Natural
Skin Care

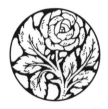

Joni Loughran's

Natural
Skin Care

Alternative & Traditional Techniques

Frog, Ltd.
Berkeley, California

Frog Ltd. Books are distributed by
North Atlantic Books
P.O. Box 12327
Berkeley, California 94712

Book and cover design by Leigh McLellan
Illustrations by Eva Googemos, Lorenzo Leissner
and Travis X. Loughran
Printed in the United States of America

Library of Congress Cataloging-in-Publication Data
Loughran, Joni.
    [Natural skin care]
    Joni Loughran's natural skin care : alternative and
traditional treatments / Joni Loughran.
        p.   cm.
    Includes bibliographical references.
    ISBN 1-883319-39-0 (trade paper)
    1. Skin—Care and hygiene.   I. Title.
RL87.L68   1995
646.7'26—dc20   95-18914

1   2   3   4   5   6   7   8   9 / 98   97   96   95

Contents

Part I Natural Skin Care Traditional Techniques

❧

2 What Is Your True Skin Type? 21

❧

3 Skin Care Treatments 29

4 Skin Care Programs 43

5 Skin Care for the Body 81

6 Natural Ingredients for Skin Care 101

7 Making Your Own Skin Care Products 111

Part II Natural Skin Care Alternative Techniques

✻

11 Color Therapy 161

✻

12 Exercise 169

✻

13 Herbal Therapy 175

✿

14 Hydrotherapy 183

✿

15 Massage 189

✿

16 Nutrition 193

17 Polarity Therapy 205

18 Reflexology 211

PART I

Natural
Skin Care

Traditional
Techniques

1

The Checklist for Beautiful Skin

1. Avoid excessive sun exposure.
2. Do not smoke.
3. Exercise regularly.
4. Get enough rest.
5. Limit your alcohol intake.
6. Use only the best cosmetics.
7. Breathe well.
8. Drink plenty of water.
9. Eat only the best foods.
10. Manage stress successfully.

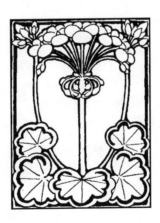

*T*he Checklist for Beautiful Skin is your most important guide for achieving and maintaining a beautiful complexion through natural skin care, bringing together the subtle and magnificent gifts of nature with the physiological facts of the skin. The result is a harmonious relationship of beautiful skin and physical/mental well-being.

An effective natural skin care program begins with understanding the factors that influence the skin's condition and appearance. Following is a detailed description of these factors. They should be evaluated individually in relation to *your* current situation. As you read through them, ask yourself, "How well am I doing compared to the optimum situation described? How can I improve?" If changes are required in your lifestyle, begin to make them *one at a time,* so that you can more easily incorporate change as a permanent condition. Once the change becomes a habit, introduce another until you have made all the improvements you want. At the end of this chapter is an evaluation and goal-setting form to help you get started.

Knowing the physical structure and function of the skin is fascinating and makes it easy to understand why skin is considered one of our most vital organs. It covers an average of eighteen square feet and weighs about seven pounds.[1,2] A cross section of the skin reveals three defined layers. The *epidermis* is the outermost layer, known as the cuticle or protective layer and is composed of tightly packed, scale-like cells which are continually being shed. An entirely new epidermis is formed approximately every twenty-eight days, a rate that seems to slow down with age. Melanin in the epidermis gives the skin its color and also protects the underlying layers from the damaging effects of the sun. The epidermis is covered with a thin layer of natural oil and perspiration that is called the acid mantle. It has an average pH of 4.5 to 5.5 and protects the skin against bacteria. Oily skin is usually less acidic; dry skin tends to be more acidic.

The layer beneath the epidermis is the *dermis,* also called the "true skin" because most vital functions of the skin are carried out there. This layer is also where the effects of age and improper care take hold. The dermis contains the glands that secrete perspiration and sebum (oil), the papilla (hair production), nerve fibers, blood vessels, lymph glands, and sense receptors. The dermis is given elasticity by the protein connective tissues called elastin and collagen, which together provide strength, resiliency, and flexibility for the skin.

Below the dermis is the third layer, called the *subcutaneous* layer, made of a fatty tissue that gives the body smoothness and contour and serves as a shock absorber and cushion for the vital organs. In addition, the subcutaneous layer stores energy and is an effective insulator. Together, these three layers—the epidermis, the dermis, and the subcutanea—form the miraculous "living fabric" known as skin.

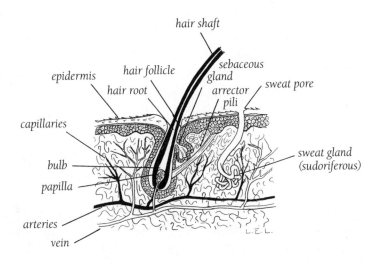

The skin maintains our health and well-being in an amazing variety of ways. In a square centimeter of skin there are one hundred sweat glands, twelve feet of nerves, hundreds of nerve endings, ten hair follicles, fifteen sebaceous glands, three feet of blood vessels, and hundreds of sensory receptors for touch, heat, and cold.[3,4] Unbroken, the skin is our first line of defense against disease and bacterial invasion. The skin regulates body temperatures, sends neurological messages to the brain, detoxifies the body by excreting wastes, breathes (takes in oxygen and releases carbon dioxide), absorbs nutrients, manufactures vitamin D, and protects the body from ultraviolet damage from the sun.

The skin, important for both our appearance and well-being, needs special care to look and perform its best. Paying attention to the items in the following checklist will help you maintain beautiful, healthy skin throughout your life.

Avoid Excessive Sun Exposure

Excessive exposure to the sun is the *number one cause* of damage and premature aging of the skin. In order to maintain youthful skin, it is necessary to spend as little time as possible in the sun, even if you are using a sunblock. Is it any wonder that the face and hands, which are almost always exposed to the sun, are the first places to show signs of aging? Peter Pugliese, M.D., a biomedical researcher who has studied the skin's response to sunlight, concluded that ninety percent of the skin problems associated with aging are the result of too much exposure to the sun. He states, "...changes produced in the skin by UVB and UVA are in the altered biochemistry of DNA, cell membrane disorders, and effects on enzymes and other proteins and amino acids."[5]

The skin undergoes a definite physiological reaction after exposure to the sun. First, the skin reddens from the dilation of blood vessels caused by the heat and light rays of the sun. Following the redness, there is increased cell production that results in a thickening of the skin. Melanin production also increases, causing the skin to darken, a response designed to provide protection against further ultraviolet harm to the body. Blisters can form and surface skin peels. Excessive sun exposure over the years results in long-term damage to the dermal layer of the skin, decreasing flexibility and elasticity while reducing the ability of collagen and elastin to support the skin and retain moisture.

Though sun exposure wreaks havoc with the complexion, it also poses health hazards. Ninety percent of all skin cancers develop on sun-exposed areas of the body and skin cancer is increasing at an alarming rate in the United States. This has been attributed to the social desirability of having a "tan" and also to atmospheric changes in the ozone layer. Dermatologists warn that no one is immune to the harmful effects of the sun but those at particularly high risk include people with fair skin, blond or red hair, and blue or green eyes. Being sensitive to the sun (such as experiencing nausea, rashes, or dizziness after exposure), having freckles, or having large or numerous moles also increases your risk. In addition, if there is a family history of melanoma or if you have suffered from a blistering sunburn anytime in your life, your risk of developing skin cancer is increased.

The Skin Cancer Foundation recommends starting sun protection in childhood, as soon as there is *any* exposure to the sun. Researchers believe that if a Sun Protection Factor (SPF) of 15 is used during the first eighteen years of life, skin cancer can be reduced by seventy-eight percent.[6] However, even when wearing a sunscreen or sunblock, people need to limit their exposure to the sun, especially those at high risk.

Guidelines for Preventing Skin Cancer and Premature Aging

1. Stay out of the sun as much as possible. Even on cloudy days, 40% to 60% of normal UV rays penetrate cloud cover.

2. Avoid extensive sun exposure between 10 A.M. and 3 P.M., even if wearing a sunblock.

3. Beware of reflected light from sand, water, cement, and snow—it can still damage the skin.

4. Wear a sunblock or sunscreen that provides both UVA and UVB protection with an SPF of at least 15 for direct sun exposure, and SPF 8 for daily, random exposure.

5. Apply sunscreen 30 minutes before going out in the sun and re-apply it every hour when swimming or perspiring. Don't forget to protect your lips and the tops of your ears.

6. For extra protection in the sun, wear clothing such as long-sleeved shirts, long-legged pants, and a sun hat. Sunglasses will help protect the skin around the eyes.

7. Avoid tanning booths and sunlamps. No matter how a tan is obtained, it is a sign of skin damage.

8. If you spend a great deal of time in the sun, have your skin thoroughly examined by a dermatologist once a year, especially if you have numerous moles.

9. At higher altitudes, sun protection needs to be increased. For every 1,000 feet of elevation, the UV rays intensify by 5%.

10. Don't wear perfumes or scents in the sun. They encourage burning and hyperpigmentation (darkened areas) on the skin.

Do Not Smoke

The *second leading cause* of skin damage and premature aging is cigarette smoking. Smoking robs the skin of its vitality and potential for being youthful and attractive. People who smoke tend to have a depleted, pallid appearance. The American Medical Association refers to this condition as "cigarette face," characterized by deep lines around the corners of the mouth, vertical lines in the upper lip, and deep lines around the eyes. The skin has a grayish cast and "tired" appearance attributed to the poor oxygen supply. This lack of oxygen leads to dehydration and dryness, causing premature wrinkling. A smoker's skin at forty years of age is similar to a non-smoker's skin at sixty years or more.[7,8] In addition, smoker's skin does not heal well or rejuvenate quickly. In fact, it is not uncommon for plastic surgeons to refuse to perform cosmetic surgery on people who smoke because of the likelihood of slow, unsuccessful healing.

Approximately 4,000 chemical compounds are produced when tobacco burns. Among those considered harmful when smoke is inhaled or comes in contact with the skin are acetone, ammonia, arsenic, benzene, carbon monoxide, formaldehyde, hydrogen cyanide, and nicotine. With cigarette smoking, carbon monoxide and nicotine impede the circulatory system, depriving the skin of much-needed oxygen and vital nutrients.

There are other unfavorable aesthetic consequences to smoking. Women who smoke at least one pack of cigarettes a day have a fifty percent greater chance of developing increased facial hair. This was discovered by researchers at the Medical College of Wisconsin and is considered related to the effects of smoking on the ovaries and/or hormonal metabolism.[9] In addition, smokers (male and female) are more likely to develop gum disease than non-smokers. In a recent study, it was found that smokers had fewer teeth with more and deeper periodontal pockets than non-smokers. Smoking is also linked to bone loss, which contributes to the loss of teeth.[10]

Although these cosmetic reasons for not smoking may appeal to vanity, smoking's ultimate curse is to overall health. Linked to a variety of health problems, smoking is the largest single cause of preventable death. It kills more than 300,000 people a year in the United States.[11] Lung diseases such as cancer, emphysema, and bronchitis can be caused by smoking. One pack of cigarettes a day, in a year's time, deposits one cup of chemical-laden tar into the lungs where it attaches to the lining. This tar cripples the lungs' natural cleansing ability. In addition, when cigarette smoke is inhaled, the air passageways become irritated and produce excess mucus which provides a breeding ground for bacteria and viruses. Smoking is also considered to be a leading cause of coronary artery disease. It damages the lining of the arteries and encourages plaque formation. Nicotine makes the heart beat faster and require more oxygen, while carbon monoxide decreases the amount of oxygen the blood can carry. This impairs the cardiovascular system, increasing the risk of heart attack. Smoking has also been linked to blood disease, ulcers, and a decline in immune function. Smoking's debilitating effect on the body worsens almost every health condition or disease. The best advice: If you don't smoke, don't start; if you *do* smoke, quit!

Exercise Regularly

There are tremendous benefits, both physical and mental, from using your body in a variety of ways and exercising to your physical capacity. A regular aerobic workout combined with flexibility and strength exercises will keep you in top physical shape and help you live a longer, healthier life. Exercise improves heart and lung function and builds resiliency and resistance to disease. It promotes weight loss and enhances the figure. Exercise improves mental health by promoting clearer thinking, increasing confidence, and reducing the effects of stress.

Exercise has been known to lift minor depression and relieve anxiety by calming the mind.

Because it contributes so much to good health and well-being, exercise is an integral part of an effective natural skin care program. Exercise aids in maintaining a clear, youthful complexion by increasing circulation which delivers the vital nutrients necessary for skin health. It also calms the nerves and promotes a deeper, more revitalizing sleep, allowing the skin to rejuvenate.

NOTE: If you have physical limitations that have discouraged you from participating in a regular exercise program, there are other forms of physical movement that may work for you. Not all of us have the endurance or abilities of athletes. Especially as we grow older, aching backs, arthritis, and stiff joints can cause problems and prevent us from taking part in more rigorous forms of exercise. But techniques such as Tai Chi, Feldenkrais, and Yoga offer easy and gentle body movements that are adaptable to almost any physical weakness. Local community centers frequently give classes in these techniques. For more information on exercise, see Chapter 12.

Get Enough Rest

Women and men lead very busy lives today—juggling the responsibilities of jobs, friends, and families. We seem to be on the go from morning until night trying to fit everything in, including an exercise program. All this activity can lead to great accomplishments and personal rewards, but it needs to be balanced with sufficient (guilt-free) rest and sleep. If not, we could suffer from the modern day malady known as "burn-out" and our complexion will suffer too.

Sleep researchers think that sleepiness has become an epidemic in this country and contributes to chronic fatigue—both mental and physical. Lack of sleep can result in poor work production, loss of concentration, and loss of creativity. People become ill-humored and dissatisfied with life. Lack of sleep is also a leading cause of car accidents.[12]

The need for sleep varies from person to person. How do you know if you are getting enough sleep? If you wake up feeling rested in the morning and don't feel sleepy until bedtime, you are most likely getting enough sleep. If it takes you more than fifteen minutes to get out of bed or if you need to set an alarm to wake up, you probably are not getting enough sleep. How to get more sleep? Go to bed earlier or try taking a cat nap during the day (as long as it doesn't disturb your evening sleep).

If you have trouble falling asleep or getting a good night's sleep, your lifestyle habits are likely contributing to the problem. Avoid sleeping late in the morning or taking naps during the day. Avoid caffeinated beverages such as coffee, green or black teas, and colas because they are stimulants. Exercising too close to bedtime can keep you awake because circulation has been revved up. Going to bed with a full stomach can also keep you awake when the digestion process is working hard. It is important to establish a regular sleep-awake pattern and practice it consistently. Your body will become accustomed to this routine and will help you sleep when you should. Sleeping well can be aided by a warm cup of herbal (relaxing) tea before bedtime, and a warm bath is especially helpful.

When you are well rested, rejuvenated, and getting enough sleep, your skin will mirror this vitality with a healthful glow.

Limit Alcohol Intake

Alcohol is an addictive drug that damages the central nervous system, the brain, and most internal organs. Potentially fatal health problems are alcohol poisoning and liver and kidney damage. Alcohol weakens the immune system and poses nutritional problems by depleting the body of vitamins and minerals. It also contains ingredients to which many people are allergic such as grains and yeast. Alcohol reduces the amount of hydrochloric acid secreted by the stomach and can cause poor digestion and absorption of food nutrients. Alcohol is also responsible for a variety of birth defects.

In the realm of skin care, alcohol prematurely ages the skin because it causes dehydration—robbing precious moisture that is necessary to keep the complexion smooth and youthful. Alcohol also impedes digestion, so vital nutrients are restricted in their ability to reach the skin. Alcohol consumption can lead to broken or distended capillaries, especially over the nose and cheeks. For good health and for a beautiful complexion, alcohol consumption should be sensibly limited.

Use Only the Best Cosmetics

The basic natural skin care program uses three types of products: a cleanser, a toner, and a moisturizer. An enhanced program adds an eye cream or oil, a mask, an exfoliant, and special nourishing treatments. Because these cosmetics are the cornerstone of every skin care program, the quality of the program depends on the quality of the cosmetics.

Cosmetics with inferior ingredients can actually harm the skin by drying it out, irritating it, or blocking the pores. Using poor-quality cosmetics may be worse than using nothing at all. Women in their thirties and forties who have rarely used skin care products often have better-looking skin than some women who experiment with every sort of commercial product that is new on the market—be it scrubs, soaps, creams, or masks. So, if you have previously neglected to care for your skin, this is the perfect time to start by following the guidelines in this chapter!

What makes high-quality cosmetics? First, read the ingredients on the product label. Does it contain anything to which you are allergic? Does it contain artificial colors or fragrances? The unfamiliar words can be confusing, so you will need to arm yourself with a book about cosmetic ingredients (such as *The Consumer's Dictionary of Cosmetic Ingredients* by Ruth Winter or *Skin Care and Cosmetic Ingredients Dictionary* by Natalia Michalun). The best cosmetics will read like a food label, with easily recognizable ingredients such as vegetable or nut oils, herbal extracts, vitamins, and aromatherapy essential oils. Surprisingly, however, you will find that some of those long, strange-looking words are acceptable ingredients from natural sources.

Next, investigate the integrity of the manufacturer and their manufacturing process. What are the company's standards? How long has it been in business? Does it have a philosophy that appeals to you? Does the company test its products on animals? Is it using quality raw ingredients that have been well formulated? Does it support its products with dependable customer service? Many times, these questions can be answered by salespeople, but ask more than one sales person to be sure the information you get is consistent. You can also contact the manufacturer directly.

There are two interesting, unorthodox ways to test cosmetics before actually using them to determine if they might be good for you. The first is with a pendulum, which can be either purchased or made by attaching a weighty object such as a ring, on a piece of string. A chain necklace with a crystal hanging from it can be used. Dangle the pendulum, holding the string between your thumb and forefinger, and when the pendulum is still, ask the question, " What is the movement for 'yes'? It should start to swing. Commonly, a "yes" swings away from you and then towards you—like a nod of the head. Or it may swing in a clockwise circle. Then, stop the pendulum and ask, "What is the movement for 'no'? This swing is often to the left and then to the right—like shaking the head. Or it may be a counter-clockwise circle. The swings for "yes" and "no" can vary for each individual, so you have to determine which is *your* signal. Then test to see if they work. Ask a question to which you already know the answer such as "Do I live in [name your town]?" The pendulum should signal yes. If this method is working for you, you can test your cosmetics. Hold the pendulum over the product and ask, "Is this product good for my skin?" You will get an answer. Pendulum work is fun and can be a helpful tool. With practice, you will become very good at it.

Muscle testing is a second unique method of testing cosmetics. You will need a partner to help you. Stand with your strongest arm straight out to the side at shoulder level. Your partner will put his or her hand on your wrist and try to push the arm down *as you resist*. This is your natural resistance strength. To check a cosmetic, put the weaker arm behind your back and have your partner put the product in your hand, without you seeing which one it is. Raise your strongest arm out to the side again (as before) and have the partner try to push it down. If the arm retains its natural resistance strength, or is stronger, the product should be good for you to use. If the arm is weaker, the product is probably not a good choice.

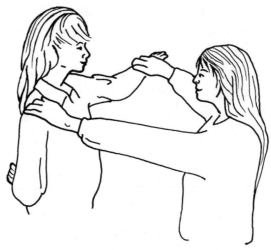

When you have set your criteria for product selection and are satisfied with the outcome of your investigations, you need to *use* the product to experience the feel, the action, and the fragrance. Some cosmetic manufacturers provide samples which allow you to try the product without a financial commitment to full sizes. An experienced salesperson or aesthetician can recommend a line of skin care products, but no one will be able to tell you unequivocally what will work the best for you. That will only be known from the experience of using it.

In general, the finest products for the best prices are available in natural food stores. This is not to say that they are *all* good—you still need to read the labels and investigate. However, there is a wide variety of products at a variety of prices, and your chances are very good for finding a product with which you will be happy.

Breathe Well

Though seldom given the credit, oxygen is our most vital nutrient. We can live for weeks without food and days without water but only a few minutes without oxygen. The art of breathing and the significance of the breath have been part of religious, philosophical, and health disciplines for thousands of years. In fact, the breath is considered to be life itself, and in many languages the words for breath and spirit are the same.

Breathing is controlled by the involuntary nervous system but is influenced by part of the voluntary nervous system such as muscles and tendons, as well as by emotions and thoughts. Breathing is the process by which waste gases (such as carbon dioxide) are eliminated from the body and fresh gases (such as oxygen) are brought in to replenish. This exchange takes place in the lungs and nutrients circulate via the bloodstream.

Most people think that breathing correctly is a natural instinct but this is not the case. Certainly we all breathe, but it is the technique and quality of breathing that make the difference, and this difference affects the quality of our lives and is reflected in the quality of our complexion.

Next time you feel anxious, check your breathing. Most likely, you will discover you are shallow breathing—using only the upper part of the lungs. At the other end of the spectrum, if you are relaxed, your breathing will be deep—using the lungs fully and slowly. By consciously breathing fully and slowly, the relaxation response can be created. This can reduce stress, which in turn benefits our health and the appearance of our skin.

Additional benefits of proper breathing are clearer thinking, increased circulation, and positive changes in moods and emotions. Proper breathing also tones the nervous system and increases energy. Particularly interesting to note is that when the breath slows, time slows, enabling us to experience life more fully.

Try this simple deep-breathing exercise. Lie on your back and slowly fill your lungs with air. Experience the expansion first in your abdomen, then the stomach, the lower lungs, and lastly, the upper lungs. To exhale, feels the abdomen "empty" first, then the stomach, and then become aware of the lungs, as the last air actually leaves them. At the end of the exhale, pause for a moment before you inhale again. Practice this technique twice a day or as often as you like. In a very short time, you will notice a change in your awareness and will experience increased relaxation.

Drink Plenty of Water

Water plays multiple fascinating roles in the human body. More than half our body weight is water, and every cell requires it to function properly. Water is involved with nearly every bodily process and is the basis of all body fluids including perspiration, blood, lymph, urine, and digestive juices. Ample water ensures that our blood purification system (circulating through the kidneys) works properly. In addition, water helps to regulate our body temperature; keeps food moving through the intestinal tract; lubricates the body's joints and mucous membranes, and transports nutrients to all parts of the body. It also provides minerals, helps to maintain muscle and skin tone, and flushes out waste material. Water benefits our skin by acting as an internal moisturizer, keeping the skin moist, supple, and clear as well as preventing premature aging.

For the average person, drinking two to three pints of clean, pure water a day is recommended. However, during illness—especially if a fever is present—more water is needed. Hot weather and vigorous exercise or work also require an increased amount. Do not wait until you are thirsty to drink water. Thirst is a response to severe dehydration. Water should be drunk throughout the day to maintain optimum internal levels.

Pure, clean, plain water is the best way to replace body fluids. Fruit juices, herbal non-diuretic teas, and vegetable juices are second best. Alcohol and caffeinated drinks are not good because they have a diuretic action, causing the body to lose water nor are heavily sugared drinks and milk recommended, as they can increase the body's need for water.

Eat Only the Best Foods

Individual nutritional needs vary depending on age, body size, gender, health, exposure to pollutants, and level of physical activity. Eating a varied diet rich in whole, natural foods, balanced in proteins, fats, and carbohydrates, and void of harmful chemicals supports a life that fulfills the physical, mental and spiritual potential of human beings. In addition, the health and beauty of the skin depends on good nutrition.

As a part of a complete natural diet, the skin especially needs plenty of water for hydration; essential fatty acids from vegetable and seed oils for suppleness, smoothness, and softness; and anti-oxidant vitamins and herbs to inhibit free-radical damage and slow the visible signs of aging. A vitamin supplementation program may be necessary for optimum nutrition. Because of our biochemical individuality, such a program will be different for everyone, and you may want to see a nutritionist to get you on the right track.

If you are experiencing any unexplained health problems or having trouble overcoming an adverse condition, you may want to be tested for hidden food allergies. You may be eating the very best natural foods but if you are overly sensitive (allergic) to them, you will not look or feel your best. Allergic reactions can take a variety of forms such as fatigue, headaches, digestive problems, mood swings, skin problems, and weakened immune function. For more information about testing for hidden food allergies call ImmunoLab, 1-800-231-9197 or Immuno Diagnostic Laboratories 707-765-6586. For more information on nutrition, see Chapter 16.

Manage Stress Successfully

There are different types of stress: mental, emotional, and physical. Emotional stress tends to take the greatest toll but stress is not all bad. In fact, life would not be very interesting if we were not met with challenges. However, too much stress—too often—with no effective and appropriate outlet, prevents the body and soul from recuperating and rejuvenating. As a result, our health as well as our complexion can suffer. Because we cannot always change the events in our lives—and isn't life full of surprises?—we must learn to change our attitude and shore up our abilities to cope. A variety of techniques have been proven helpful. Meditation, creative visualization, and counseling can ease the tension. Proper breathing, massage, and regular exercise are beneficial. Getting more sleep, improving the diet and pursuing spiritual interests also help people deal with stress. It is comforting to remember that everyone's life is stressful at one time or another. It is a shared human experience and we have each other to help. For more information on stress, see Chapter 19.

Evaluation and Goal Setting

How are you doing?	Great	OK	Not So Good
1. Avoiding sun exposure.	☐	☐	☐
2. Not smoking.	☐	☐	☐
3. Exercising regularly.	☐	☐	☐
4. Getting enough rest.	☐	☐	☐
5. Limiting alcohol.	☐	☐	☐
6. Using the best cosmetics.	☐	☐	☐
7. Breathing well.	☐	☐	☐
8. Drinking plenty of water.	☐	☐	☐
9. Eating healthful, natural food.	☐	☐	☐
10. Managing stress successfully.	☐	☐	☐

List those items that were checked "Not So Good" in order of importance to you and describe how you can improve.

1.

2.

3.

4.

5.

6.

7.

8.

9.

10.

List those items that were checked "OK" in order of importance to you and describe how you can improve.

1.

2.

3.

4.

5.

6.

7.

8.

9.

10.

Now, set your goals. List below the first item that you are going to work to improve, the second, the third, and so on until you have listed everything in your OK and Not So Great lists. When you begin working on your first item, write in the date. When you have completed it, record that date, put a check-mark and congratulate yourself! Then move on to your second item, until you have completed your list. Good Luck!

1.

2.

3.

4.

5.

6.

7.

8.

9.

10.

2

What Is Your True Skin Type?

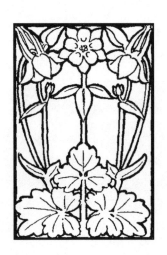

A basic physiological description of human skin is the same for everyone. The skin is our largest vital organ and our first line of defense against bacterial invasion. Yet, from person to person there are characteristic differences that result from heredity, lifestyle, or age. These differences classify one's skin as a certain "type." For example, the English tend to have sensitive skin; people who are out in the sun a lot usually have dry, dehydrated skin; and teenagers frequently have oily or blemished skin.

It is important to identify your true skin type so you will be able to select the correct skin care products and know what special guidelines to follow. Read the following descriptions and find the one that most closely portrays your skin.

Normal Skin

Normal skin is the goal of every skin care program. Yet, it may be that the only truly normal skin is that of a child, when the skin is velvety smooth and soft, taut, resilient, and free of wrinkles or blemishes. After childhood, the skin goes through many stages and changes significantly over time.

For our purposes in "skin typing," normal skin indicates that the water and oil glands on the face are producing just the right amount to hydrate (add moisture) and protect the skin (prevent moisture loss). Normal skin's appearance is moist, plump and dewy. The pores are small to medium in size. There are few or no blemishes and minimal sun-damage. The skin is of medium thickness and has an even tone. Normal skin is soft, smooth and firm with good elasticity. It may have some oiliness in the "T zone" (the forehead, nose, and chin), but unless the oil is excessive, the skin is still considered normal. *Key description: Balanced*

Oily Skin

Oily skin has sebaceous (oil) glands that are too active. The pores are visibly more noticeable than in other skin types and are medium to large in size. Oily skin has a shiny appearance and is usually thicker, firmer, and less sensitive than the other types. Oily skin appears most often among those aged twelve to twenty-two, but some people may have oily skin all their lives, although it should gradually become less oily with age. While there is a tendency for clogged pores, blackheads, and blemishes, the good news for oily skin is that it usually has a youthful appearance and does not show the signs of aging as quickly as the other skin types. *Key description: Overactive*

Dry Skin

Dry skin has a lack of oil, a lack of water, or both. Skin that is lacking in oil is called simple dry skin. Skin that is lacking in water is called dehydrated skin. If the skin is thin and the pores are barely visible, it is probably lacking in oil (and possibly water as well). If the skin is thick with visible pores but has the characteristics of dry skin, it is probably only lacking water.

Dry skin can be seen in people of all ages. Women tend to have drier skin than men, and fair-skinned people have dry skin more often than dark-skinned people. Dry skin can feel tight and may have visible flaking. It is often delicate, easily irritated, and usually sensitive to cold weather. Dry skin has a matte finish with no sheen and can have a rough feel to it.

Simple dry skin (lacking oil) for the younger woman has the advantages of a fine texture and clear complexion. But as that woman ages, her skin will develop fine lines and will wrinkle sooner than the other skin types.

Many people think that they have dry skin when they actually have a superficial dry condition. Superficial dryness is caused by exposure to the sun, sea air, wind, or pollutants. It is also caused by improper skin-care habits such as using soap as a cleanser or not using a moisturizer for protection. These factors contribute to the skin becoming dehydrated and dry. A well-designed skin care program that eliminates the causes of superficial dryness will also eliminate the symptoms, and the skin's moisture content on the outermost layer can be restored. *Key description: Underactive*

NOTE: The symptoms of certain skin diseases such as eczema, mild psoriasis, or atopic dermatitis are sometimes mistaken for dry skin.

Combination Skin

Combination skin refers to skin with two or more distinctly different characteristics on different parts of the face. The most common combination skin is oily in certain areas and then dry or normal in the other areas. Usually, the "T-zone" (forehead, nose, and chin) is oily and the cheeks and around the eyes are normal or dry. Ninety-five percent of combination skin types will fit this description. The other five percent can have a variety of combinations such as a blemished forehead, dry cheeks and normal everywhere else, or the skin could be normal in the "T-zone" and dry everywhere else. Combination skin can be seen in people of all ages but most typically in those aged twelve to forty. *Key description: Asymmetric*

Sensitive Skin

Sensitive skin is characterized by overreaction to external influences. It is easily irritated by certain cosmetics, handling, and environmental factors (such as sun, wind, and temperature extremes). Exposure can result in redness, a rash, itching, stinging, or burning. Sensitive skin has a tendency to develop distended or broken capillaries as well as allergies, and it usually sunburns easily.

Sensitivity can be present in normal, dry, and oily skins and at any age. However, it is most common among people of Celtic descent, particularly redheads and people with blond hair and blue eyes. Sensitive skin is thinner than other skin types, and the nerve endings and blood vessels are closer to the surface which is thought to be one of the causes of the oversensitivity.

Sensitive skin needs to be treated gently. The causes of irritation can vary with each individual, so a sensitive skin care program can also vary. Generally, however, products that contain alcohol, artificial colors, and artificial fragrances should be avoided. Highly active ingredients such as aromatherapy essential oils or alpha hydroxy acids may also need to be avoided. Preservatives have also been known to cause problems for some people. *Key description: Delicate*

Blemished Skin

Blemished skin is characterized by chronic pustules, blackheads, whiteheads, and sometimes scarring. Blemished skin is most common during the teenage years, but it is not uncommon to find this condition in adults. Teenage skin is prone to blemishes because of the increase in hormone production, which stimulates oil glands in the skin. If the oil flows freely from the pore, blemishes will not develop and the skin will simply be an "oily" skin type. However, this overproduction of oil often combines with a build-up of dead skin cells and clogs the pore. As pressure builds, leakage into the surrounding tissue occurs. Bacteria flourish in the clogged pore and the surrounding inflamed tissue, resulting in an infection and a blemish. Adult blemishes are usually attributed to factors such as general health, diet, stress, air pollution, and reactions to cosmetics. They can also be the result of illness, poor systemic elimination, disrupted intestinal flora, hereditary influences, and hidden food allergies. (See Chapter 1, "The Checklist for Beautiful Skin: Eat Only the Best Foods.")

It is important for people with blemishes to know that blemished skin (or acne) is not a "normal" condition. It is a symptom of physical imbalance. Because the causes of the problem differ, there is no *one* cure that works for everyone. A blemished skin condition may stem from a deep-rooted systemic imbalance, a superficial systemic problem, or external causes. Mainstream medicine's chief weapon against acne is drug therapy such as antibiotics and Accutane (a vitamin A derivative). Because long term use of antibiotics generally weakens the immune system and disrupts the intestinal flora, and Accutane has been shown to cause birth defects, natural methods of controlling blemishes are preferred.[1] An integrated program of appropriate skin care, skin care products, diet, and lifestyle habits *can* be successful, but it takes more time than the short-term successes of drug therapy. It also takes dedication, commitment, and discipline. Guidance from naturopathic physicians, nutritionists, and skin care professionals can be a great help and is recommended for those seeking a natural, healthy, long-term solution to chronic blemishes. *Key description: Congested and upset*

Aging Skin

"Aging" is a characteristic that may be combined with any of the other skin types—for example, aging/sensitive skin or aging/blemished skin, or it can simply mean mature skin. When the aging condition is present, it may be appropriate for the individual, or it may be "premature." Appropriate aging occurs naturally from the passage of time and the slowing down of the glandular functions in the skin lessening its ability to rejuvenate. Premature aging is the result of overexposure to the sun (the number one cause), smoking, improper skin care, mistreatment, poor lifestyle habits, or health problems. In these cases, the skin looks older than it should.

Visible signs of aging usually develop by the age of thirty, when cellular turnover starts to slow down, making the skin look dull and less vibrant. Laugh lines and fine furrows begin to show. By the time we are forty, the pigment cells and immune cells in the skin—our protection against the hazards of the sun—decrease, making our skin more prone to sun damage. At this age, the skin also may be showing signs of sagging due to weakened elasticity. Expression lines deepen, and discolorations or "age spots" are common. When we are fifty, the oil glands significantly slow down. This decrease in oil production causes dryness, especially in cold, dry, or wintry climates. As time goes by, these accumulating factors continue creating the lines and wrinkles, the dryness and the roughness, and the poor elasticity and sagging that are common signs of aging skin.

Though the skin cannot be prevented from aging, *premature* aging is completely avoidable. In addition, healthy living and natural skin care techniques can rejuvenate even the most tired complexions. *Key description: Inactive*

Determining Your Skin Type

After reading the above descriptions, you probably have a good idea what type of skin you have. But before you decide, consider your heritage. Different atmospheres and weather conditions all over the world affect skin characteristics, both individual and heredity. Extreme climates—both hot and cold—tend to produce thicker-skinned people. Hot climates produce people with more color and more oil in the skin. People from moist, cool climates usually have thin, dry, sensitive skin. Generally speaking, Caucasian skin can be fair (Nordic or British) or olive (Mediterranean). Fair skin is light in color, has a thin texture, and is vulnerable to dryness and damage from the environment. Olive skin tends to be oilier and less vulnerable to damage. Black skin has high concentrations of melanin and is usually more oily than dry. Hispanic skin is usually normal to oily with more melanin than Caucasian skin.

After reading the descriptions and considering your heritage, use your sight and touch to make a final analysis. This should be done in the morning. The evening before, wash and rinse your face thoroughly with a very mild soap (this *one* time only!). Do not apply any moisturizer or night creams. Upon arising, take a sheet of tissue paper and hold it against your face. Then examine the tissue paper. Are there oil marks on it? In what areas? Take a close look at your skin in the mirror with natural light. What do the pores look like? Is the skin shiny or dull in appearance? Correlate this information with the descriptions of the basic skin types.

Next, use your sense of touch. Does the skin feel rough or tight? Does it have an oily feel to it? In which areas? Make a note of your findings. Then, rinse your face with warm water and pat it dry.

It is best if you can take a second and third accounting of the skin during the day. Do not apply any moisturizer or make-up. A few hours after the first look, examine your skin again with sight and touch. Rinse and pat dry, and then check one more time a few hours later. This analysis will give you a good idea of how much and where your skin is producing oil.

Once you have determined your skin type, keep in mind that your skin is always in a state of transition and can change significantly. This means that periodically you will need to re-evaluate your skin. Transitions might be the result of your skin care program improving your skin, different environmental conditions, your diet, general health, stress level, or the aging process. Although you may have normal skin today, after years pass, it will probably become dry. It is not uncommon for people with oily skin in their youth to develop normal skin as they grow older. Damaged and superficially dry skin can recapture its vitality with proper care and become more normal. You may even notice a difference in your skin with the turn of the seasons. These changes need to be identified, as they determine the skin's immediate condition and affect the design of your skin care program.

3

Skin Care Treatments

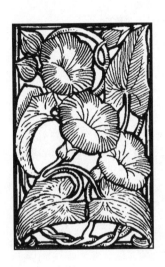

*A*fter identifying your skin type as described in Chapter 2, the next step is to become acquainted with the treatments and the types of products that will make up your natural skin care program. At the foundation of every program for all skin types are four simple steps: compressing, cleansing, toning, and moisturizing. Special treatments enhance the program and can produce dramatic benefits for the skin. These treatments include steams, exfoliants, aromatherapy treatments, masks, eye creams and facial misters. A variety of products is available for both the basic steps and the special treatments. (For guidelines in selecting quality products, see Chapter 1, "The Checklist for Beautiful Skin: Use Only the Best Cosmetics.")

Basic Skin Care Treatments

Compressing

The first step is to pre-cleanse the skin using a treatment called "facial compressing." This is an important part of the program because it begins to soften and loosen soil and dirt—making the cleansing process easier and more effective. Warm water compresses relax the face, encourage glandular activity, and increase circulation while hydrating the skin. Cool water compresses are refreshing, have a toning effect, calm inflammation and also hydrate the skin. Essential oils can be added to the water for compressing, contributing the benefits of aromatherapy in this pre-cleansing step. See Chapter 9 for more information on using essential oils in compresses and other ways.

How to Compress

❧ Thoroughly rinse a clean washcloth or cloth diaper to remove any detergent residue. (Bacteria will begin to grow quickly on a used washcloth, so use a clean one every day.)

❧ Fill the basin with cool, tepid, or warm water depending on your skin type. (Normal: cool to warm, Oily: cool to tepid, Dry: warm, Combination: warm, Sensitive: tepid to warm, Blemished: cool to tepid, Mature: warm)

❀ Lean over the basin, dip the washcloth in the water and hold the washcloth to your face and neck for a few moments.

❀ Repeat the dipping and applying process for at least 10 compresses.

❀ Cleanse as usual.

NOTE: Avoid extreme water temperatures on the face. *Hot* water is drying because it strips away the natural skin oils and can also prompt small capillaries to swell and possibly break—causing small red lines to appear. *Cold* water can harm the tiny capillaries as well and can suppress glandular functions in the skin.

Cleansing

The next step is thorough cleansing to remove the soil and debris that collect on the surface of the skin. This includes make-up, dirt, dust, waste products excreted by the skin, and dead skin cells. If cleansing is done properly and with the right product, it will help to prevent problems such as clogged pores, blemishes, skin irritations, and premature aging. The best cleanser for you will clean away make-up and dirt without leaving the skin dehydrated, irritated, or stripped of its natural oils. There are two rules of thumb for cleansing that apply for all types of skin and every age group: *Never use soap and always treat your skin gently.*

Your choice of cleanser will depend on your type of skin and your preference for the feel, smell, and performance of the product. Cleansers come in four basic forms: creams, milks, gels, and foaming cleansers. Cream cleansers are heavy and thick and contain more oil than water. Milky cleansers are a balanced formulation of oil and water and are lighter and more fluid than cream. Gels are usually oil-free and have a thickened, gel-like consistency. Foaming cleansers contain ingredients that create suds. There are some foaming cleansers available now that do not contain harsh detergents or soap, a natural alternative for those who like their cleanser to have a foaming action.

Recommended Cleansers by Skin Type

Normal: Oil-free cleansing gel, cleansing milk, or soap-free foaming cleanser

Oily:	*Younger skin*—oil-free cleansing gel.
	Older skin—oil-free cleansing gel or cleansing milk
Dry:	Cleansing milk or cleansing cream
Combination:	Use the recommended cleanser for the skin type of each area, or choose one cleanser for the entire face that is good for the drier area. It is less harmful to the skin to under-clean an oily area than over-clean a dry area.
Sensitive:	Cleansing milk or cleansing cream.
Blemished:	*Younger skin*—oil-free cleansing gel. *Older skin*—oil-free cleansing gel or well-formulated cleansing milk.
Mature:	Cleansing milk or cleansing cream.

How to Use a Cleanser

After compressing, apply your cleanser to dampened skin (face and neck) using a patting and pressing action. Apply as if you were hugging your skin with your fingers and palms of your hands. You may move around the skin in soft, gentle circles but do not scrub and do not use heavy pressure that might weaken the underlying support structure or force impurities into the skin. Work in this manner for about two minutes and then rinse, rinse, rinse with warm water until the cleanser has been completely removed. Follow with a cool-water splash and then pat your skin with a towel to remove excess water. Do not pat completely dry.

The Soap Controversy

Soap and products that contain soap or harsh detergents are *not* an option as facial cleansers because they are too strong. They are very alkaline and destroy the skin's protective acid mantle as well as strip the skin of its natural oils. The regular use of soap or detergent contributes to the premature aging of the skin because of the drying action. Dr. Peter Pugliese, dermatologist and author of *Advanced Professional Skin Care* (APSC Publishing, 1991), states, "Using soap as the major facial cleansing agent has serious drawbacks. To what extent it adds to wrinkle formation has not been determined exactly, but there is no doubt that it is a contributing agent."

Be certain to read the labels of cleansers and avoid those that contain soap or detergent. (Hint: if your cleanser is leaving your face "squeaky clean," it is too strong.)

Toning

The third step is the toner, which is used after the skin has been cleansed, thoroughly rinsed, and patted damp-dry. A good toner will remove any residue left by the cleanser—acting as a second-step cleanser—without causing dryness. It should also reestablish the acid pH of the skin (if it has been disrupted by the cleanser). Toners condition the skin as well as prepare the skin for the next step, which is moisturizing.

The toners that were available many years ago were poorly formulated and usually contained alcohol which not only removed every bit of cleanser but every bit of natural skin oil as well. These toners were too drying and often irritating. Today, toners have been improved and most no longer contain alcohol. Look for toners designed for your skin type with simple, natural ingredients such as aloe, herbal extracts, and aromatherapy hydrosols.

How to Use a Toner

Saturate a cotton ball and then *gently wipe* the face and neck. Do not scrub and do not apply around the eyes or the mouth because these areas are prone to dryness. Using a cotton ball is more effective than just patting the toner on the face because the cotton ball will lift off and take away any residue or remaining soil. Some very dry or sensitive skins may not be able to use a toner at all.

Moisturizing

Moisturizing is the final step of the basic skin care routine. All skin types benefit from the hydration and protection that a moisturizer provides, though some skin types need it more than others. Moisturizers are most effective when applied after the skin has been hydrated by water from a shower, bath, facial compresses, or facial misting. Using a moisturizer serves two purposes. First, it forms a protective barrier that prevents moisture loss and guards the skin against the effects of harsh weather and environmental conditions. (A well-formulated moisturizer will do this without clogging the pores.) Second, a good moisturizer will contain effective humectants (such as glycerin or hyaluronic acid) that hold moisture next to the skin to counteract dryness and help prevent the signs of aging. Moisturizers can make the skin feel softer and smoother while nurturing it with active ingredients such as vitamins, herbal extracts, and essential oils.

Moisturizers tend to be the most elaborate of the three basic skin care products and the most expensive. They have a smooth, creamy consistency and are usually emulsions (combinations) of water and oil, a design that imitates our natural skin protection system (sweat and oil glands excrete water and oil on the surface of the skin.) The "richer" moisturizers have more oil than water and provide a heavier protective barrier. The "lighter" ones have more water and are more hydrating but do not give as much protection. To know whether or not the moisturizer you are using provides enough protection, you should be able to feel that it is still there two or three hours after applying. If you cannot and your skin feels dry, then you need a richer moisturizer.

Some moisturizers are formulated as night creams and others as day creams. Generally, the difference is that night creams contains more active, nourishing ingredients to rejuvenate the skin while you sleep. The day creams are designed to be more protective because of the day-time exposure to the environment. Not all manufacturers make both a day and night cream, and there is a difference of opinion about the use of and need for having two types. Some companies believe that one cream is sufficient for both situations. Others claim it is important to sleep with the face clean so that it can breathe. Still others feel that night is the time to nurture the skin with special ingredients. This may ultimately be a matter of personal choice. However, if you choose to use a night cream, use it sparingly. A thick coat of cream prevents the skin from breathing and excreting properly while you are sleeping.

How to Use a Moisturizer

Choose a moisturizer designed for your skin type, and follow these guidelines. First, moisturize only *when* and *where* you need it. In some cases, when a moisturizer is applied to skin that does not need oil, it can cause congestion or blemishes. Use your moisturizer with discretion. The areas that are tight or dry are the areas that need a moisturizer. Second, the type of moisturizer you are using may need to be changed with the seasons or with a change of environment. If you are in extreme cold with winds, you need a richer, heavier moisturizer for increased protection, and you may need to apply it where you normally do not. If it is summer and you are in humid weather, you may only need a moisturizer on your cheeks. Exercise flexibility when using a moisturizer, depending on your skin type and the situation. Lastly, moisturizers should be applied with a patting, pressing, and smoothing technique. Avoid dragging or stretching the skin.

Special Skin Care Treatments

Mother Nature has given us a remarkable collection of safe, healthy, and effective ways to have a beautiful complexion. Discussed below are steaming treatments to super-cleanse and hydrate; exfoliants to rid the skin of dead skin cell build-up; aromatherapy treatments to rejuvenate; masks to condition and deep-cleanse; eye creams to protect; and facial misting to hydrate and refresh. These special treatments are a powerful addition to the basic steps (compressing, cleansing, toning, moisturizing) and are recommended to complete your natural skin care program.

Steaming

Facial steaming serves a number of purposes for skin care. The warm, moist vapor hydrates the skin, temporarily softening fine lines and wrinkles. It increases circulation, thereby increasing the oxygen and nutrient supply, and encouraging cellular rejuvenation. Steaming encourages the pores to clean from within, eliminating toxins. It also softens dead surface skin cells as well as oil, make-up, and dirt residue so that it can be more effectively cleansed. When used in conjunction with facial masks, steaming will increase the mask's effectiveness.

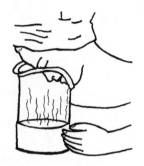

Small facial steaming machines are available for home use from drug and department stores and are relatively inexpensive. The face-over-the-pot method is not recommended because it does not provide a continuous, gentle steam with a consistent temperature. The small facial steamers are much safer and more effective.

While everybody's skin can benefit from steaming, there are guidelines for each type. Begin with a clean face and protect the delicate area around the eyes with an eye cream and protect the lips with a lip balm during the steaming process. If you have "broken" capillaries (couperose) on your face, this area should also be protected before steaming. In this case, use a rich moisturizer.

Recommended Steaming Time

Normal:	Steam once a week for 8-10 minutes.
Oily:	Steam once or twice a week for 8-10 minutes.
Dry:	Frequent steaming is not appropriate and could cause dryness and irritation. However, once or twice a month will help to hydrate the skin. Steam only for 2-5 minutes, at enough distance from the steam source that it does not feel hot.
Combination:	Follow the guidelines for the predominant skin type.
Sensitive:	Frequent steaming is not appropriate and could cause dryness and irritation. However, once or twice a month will help to hydrate the skin. Steam only for 2-3 minutes, at enough distance from the steam source that it does not feel hot.
Blemished:	Steam once or twice a week for 8-10 minutes to encourage the skin to self-cleanse and to unclog pores. The steam should be warm and gentle—not too hot.
Mature:	Frequent steaming is not appropriate and could cause dryness. However, once or twice a month will help to hydrate the skin and stimulate circulation. Steam only for 2-5 minutes, at enough distance from the steam source that it does not feel hot.

After you have steamed your face for the appropriate amount of time, rinse with warm water. If the steaming has softened and loosened a lot of debris, it is best to cleanse the face again with your facial cleanser. Then splash with cool water and pat dry.

Exfoliants

Exfoliants have been used in skin care for many years. Their purpose is to encourage the removal of dead cells and debris from the surface of the skin, revealing a softer, smoother complexion. In the past, the most common exfoliants were rough sponges or products with a grainy texture, called "scrubs." Many of these products were poorly designed or formulated and were so rough that they scratched and damaged the skin. Sharp-edged nut shells were often included in the ingredients. In some cases, these products were carelessly recommended for blemished skin which not only could aggravate the blemishes, but also spread the infection. The consumer was poorly educated in the use of sponge and scrub-type exfoliants, and the result was more skin damage than improvement. Today, better scrubs are available that use gentler particles for texture such as oatmeal, almond flour or jojoba beads.

Green papaya and alpha hydroxy acids are two new types of exfoliants which are a boon to natural skin care. They are very effective for improving the look and feel of the skin—far more effective than the granular exfoliants. They can be used by all skin types except the most sensitive and are especially beneficial for sun-damaged and aging skin. Both are being formulated in masks, liquid treatments, moisturizers, and lotions. Green papaya is the enzyme in papaya fruit before it ripens. The green papaya digests "dead" protein (dead skin cells) with an enzyme called *papain* and makes the skin feel softer and smoother. Green papaya is gentle yet effective and can, if properly formulated, be used by most sensitive skin and also around the eyes. Alpha hydroxy acids are derived from a variety of sources. Malic acid is derived from apples; citric acid comes from lemons, limes, and oranges; glycolic acid is from sugar cane; tartaric acid comes from wine grapes; and lactic acid comes from sour milk. Alpha hydroxy acids exfoliate the skin by dissolving a glue-like protein substance that holds dead skin cells together on the surface of the skin. Regular and consistent use of alpha hydroxy acids, in the correct dilution, results in the exfoliation of these skin cells, revealing smoother, softer skin, improved texture, and a reduction in fine lines and wrinkles. Alpha hydroxy acids have also been known to help prevent blemishes as well as improve existing blemished conditions.

Aromatherapy Treatments

Aromatherapy uses essential oils from aromatic plants for the purpose of restoring or enhancing health and beauty. Aromatherapy has been used in one form or another throughout history by people all over the world. Essential oils are highly concentrated, volatile oils found in tiny droplets between the cells of the plant. They are responsible for the fragrance of a plant, in fact the term aromatherapy literally means "fragrant remedy."

Aromatherapy treatments seem to appeal to everyone. Not only are they wonderful for the body, they are also wonderful for the psyche. Essential oils have been found to influence the emotions because as they are inhaled through the nose, the aroma travels to a part of the brain that controls memories and emotions. Essential oils can also stimulate natural chemicals in the brain that are responsible for feelings of pleasure.

Essential oils are a delight to use in skin care treatments because of their enticing fragrances and their profound effect. They are a marvelous way to pamper the skin, and virtually all types of skin can benefit. The effectiveness of essential oils is due to their ability to penetrate the skin. They have a small and simple molecular structure, and when applied to the skin, they pass into the dermal layer where they can truly affect the skin's condition. The benefits commonly associated with essential oils include rejuvenating, balancing, and calming. The most familiar essential oils used in cosmetics are from flowers such as lavender, chamomile, and rose. These oils are formulated into many skin care products such as facial oils, cleansers, toners, moisturizers, masks, and misters, where their benefits can be gained and one's complexion improved. All of these products are available commercially, but you can also make some of them yourself from the recipes in Chapter 7 of this book.

See Chapter 9 for more details about aromatherapy, including a list of the most popular cosmetic essential oils, their role in skin care, their effect on the psyche, and practical ways to use them.

Masks

Facial masks can be used by all skin types, depending on the formulation. Masks are formulated in a variety of ways for different purposes. They are used to moisturize, tighten, cleanse, soothe, stimulate, exfoliate, or nourish the skin.

Clay-based masks are tightening and cleansing because of the clay's ability to absorb oil and toxins. Clay tones and refreshes the skin while its action stimulates surface circulation. Some clays are very high in minerals which provide nourishment to the skin. Commercial clay masks are often formulated with additional ingredients such as herbs, essential oils, or vitamins that combine well with clay. Because clay masks can be slightly drying, they are recommended for people with normal skin (twice a month) or with oily or problem skin (once a week). They are not recommended for dry or mature skin unless they have been formulated with ingredients that counteract the drying effects.

Cream masks are designed to soothe, moisturize, and nourish the skin. Cream masks stimulate surface circulation and are especially good for dry, sun-damaged, aging, or sensitive skin. Depending on the formulation, they can be used about once a week. Normal skin will also benefit from cream masks, particularly when it feels drier than usual as a result of environmental exposure or change of the season.

Eye Creams

Eye creams are designed to protect and nurture the delicate skin around the eyes. Because this area has few oil glands and because the eyes are constantly moving, this is usually the first place to show signs of age. Eye creams are designed to prevent this from happening prematurely. The formulation of an eye cream must take into consideration that the eye area loses moisture easily but that it cannot tolerate heavy creams. Too rich a cream can cause whiteheads or other clogged-pore problems. Eye creams are available in formulations ranging from lightweight oils to heavy creams. Eye gels are also available. Personal preference should be your guide, but keep in mind that the eye area is sensitive so product ingredients should be gentle and contain NO artificial colors or fragrances.

People of all skin types should begin using an eye treatment around the age of twenty-five or sooner if necessary. Even people with oily or problem skin can use this "special treatment" although they should use the lighter formulas. Eye creams, oils, and gels should be applied sparingly around the eye in a pat-and-press method. Do not rub or stretch the skin. Using too much product or getting product in the eye can cause puffiness. Eye treatments can be worn during the day and at night while you sleep. The lighter eye treatments are better during the day to avoid disrupting eye make-up. The heavier ones are excellent at night after you have hydrated your skin with facial compresses, cleansing, and rinsing.

If you experience *occasional* eye puffiness or discoloration, there are a variety of causes. It may be due to lack of sleep or to illness. Hangovers can also cause these problems. Whatever the reason, the following home remedies can help minimize it. Place cold cucumber slices over closed eyes for about fifteen minutes while lying down. This has a cooling, soothing and healing effect. Dip cotton balls in cold milk, squeeze out the excess liquid and use the same as the cucumber slices. Acupressure used around the eyes can help drain the fluids and reduce puffiness. (For more information, see Chapter 8, "Acupressure."

Facial Misting

Facial misting is an enjoyable and refreshing skin care treatment. Facial misters are bottles with a pump sprayer. The contents can be plain water or a special blend of water with herbal extracts, essential oils, aloe vera, floral waters, or hydrosols. The primary function of a facial mister is to hydrate the skin. Facial dryness, including fine lines, can be reduced with regular facial misting. However, in order for misters to be effective, they should be used in conjunction with a

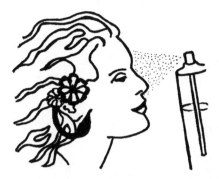

moisturizer that contains a good humectant. The mister should emit a very fine spray so that it will not disturb make-up. Facial misting is good for all skin types, especially dry and aging, and can be used as often as desired. It is recommended at least three times a day—morning, noon, and night and is especially important in dry climates, air-conditioned rooms, and airplanes, where there is little moisture in the air. (Care should be taken not to get the misting liquid in the eyes, especially if you are using one that contains essential oils. This could be irritating to the eyes.)

4

Skin Care Programs

Guidelines for Normal, Oily, Dry, Combination, Sensitive, Blemished, & Mature/Aging Skin

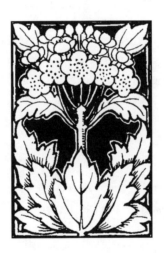

*T*he following guidelines will help you begin a daily, weekly and monthly skin care program based on your skin type. The guidelines include the basic steps (such as cleansing and toning), special treatments (such as exfoliation, masks and misting), and a suggested routine. There are also special considerations to increase the effectiveness of your program. The guidelines for blemished skin include "Alternative Techniques for Blemished Skin," which have proven to be immensely helpful in correcting a blemished skin condition. If you follow these guidelines, combined with the information from Chapter 1, "The Checklist for Beautiful Skin," your complexion will improve and look its best!

Seasonal Considerations

Our complexion is affected by the environment and the weather. Just as nature slows during autumn's passage into winter and comes alive again during the spring and summer, the skin reflects this cyclical pattern. Taking the seasons into consideration as part of your skin care program is important to maintain a truly effective routine.

Winter

Depending on where you live, winter can be an extreme season with cold wind, rain, and snow. Harsh weather can cause your skin to become dry, flaky, rough, chapped and irritated. Small capillaries on the face can be damaged—showing up as tiny, red, spidery lines. Sebaceous glands are slowed down by the cold and produce less oil, so the skin is less protected and does not retain moisture as efficiently. Most skin is affected by the wintry elements but sensitive, dry, and mature skins are particularly susceptible.

In the winter, your skin is exposed to the low temperatures and dry air outdoors, combined with warm indoor air that is artificially heated. Both of these conditions dry the skin, and the effect is made worse by going in and out, exposing the skin to both temperature extremes.

Though winter conditions cannot be avoided, your skin care routine can help to counteract them. During the winter months, use gentle cleansers and moisturize well. If you are going to be directly exposed to the wind or snow or extreme cold, use a heavier, "richer" moisturizer than usual. Be sure to include an eye cream. Wearing a sunblock of SPF 15 is still necessary because UV damage is always a risk. Avoid saunas and steam rooms because they cause the skin to lose valuable moisture. Stay away from tanning booths too—they damage the skin.

The skin should be protected with clothing such as hats, scarves, and gloves during the winter, and whenever your hands are exposed to water, apply hand cream. Keep the skin away from extreme hot and cold water temperatures, and protect the lips often with a lip balm. Avoid licking your lips—it causes chapping. Drink plenty of water to keep the skin moisturized from within. Take fewer or shorter baths and showers and moisturize the entire body afterwards. Use humidifiers in artificially heated rooms to put moisture back in the air. Wintertime may increase your need for dietary oil. Canola, flax seed, olive, and sunflower are particularly good. Exfoliation is still important during the winter but care must be taken. If the skin is irritated from the weather, exfoliation may cause further irritation.

Spring

Spring is the time for the skin to normalize from the winter cold. All of nature begins to wake up from a long winter's rest, and so does the skin. Spring-time weather isn't too hot or too cold and the skin reflects this by normalizing—not being oilier or drier than usual. During the spring, the skin is recovering from winter exposure. Because the air is warmer and has more moisture in it, you can start using a lighter moisturizer than the one you may have used during the winter. Sun protection, as always, needs to be maintained.

Summer

Protecting the skin from the sun is the main skin care issue of the summer months. Review Chapter 1, "The Checklist for Beautiful Skin: Avoid Excessive Sun Exposure." Wear your sunblock regularly and don't forget to include the tops of your ears, your lips, and the backs of your hands. Keep a sunblock in your purse and your car so that you are never without it during this season. Provide additional protection for the eye area by wearing large sunglasses that block UV rays. A broad-brimmed hat is also helpful.

Though sun exposure is a concern, the warmer temperatures of summer are easier on the skin than cold winter temperatures. Glandular activities in the skin are stimulated by the heat, which is great for dry and mature skin.

Your skin care routine should emphasize facial misting during this season to keep the skin cool and hydrated. Body misting is beneficial and enjoyable, too. Keep a mister in the refrigerator for a refreshing experience! Cleanse and tone as usual, but you may need to change your moisturizer to a lighter formula. Stay away from overly oily or greasy products. Be sure to drink plenty of water to replace what is lost through perspiration during these hotter months.

Autumn

Autumn is a time for the skin to normalize, as all of nature begins to slow down for the winter. The weather isn't too hot or too cold, and the skin also reflects this by not being oilier or drier, just as in the spring. Recovering from summer exposure is the focus for autumn skin care. The skin may require additional exfoliation to get rid of the surface skin cells damaged by the summer sun and outdoor activities. The skin may be flaking or peeling. Green papaya, alpha hydroxy acids, and dry brush massage are excellent for removing the dry, dead skin cells.

Cleanse as usual, and if you are experiencing flakiness, you may want to avoid using a toner until the skin has returned to a normal healthy state. In addition, because the air is cooling, it is becoming drier. If you changed your moisturizer to a lighter formula during the summer, you may need to replace it with a heavier one. Continue drinking plenty of water and start using a humidifier if you have begun to use the heater in your home or at work.

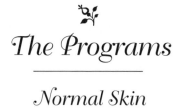

The Programs

Normal Skin

Characteristics: *smooth, firm, moisture-balanced,*
oil-balanced, medium pores, soft and unwrinkled

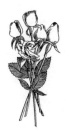

The skin care program for normal skin is designed to *maintain* its well-balanced state with proper care and to *prevent* premature aging. "Normal" is the condition that all other skin types are trying to achieve, and the truth is, after childhood it is rare that the skin is ever truly "normal" again. See Part II to learn how to benefit normal skin using alternative techniques.

The Steps for Normal Skin

Compressing: Use cool or warm compresses. (For more information, see Chapter 3, "Skin Care Treatments," under "Compressing.")

Cleansing: Normal skin is the only skin type that can use the widest variety of cleansers such as oil-free, milky, or soap-free foaming cleansers. Oil-free cleansers are good for younger, normal skin (teen age to twenty years old), and the milky cleansers are good for older normal skin (early twenties).

Normal skin can be cleansed twice a day—in the morning and before going to sleep. As it matures, however, normal skin will become drier. When this occurs, cleansing should be reduced to once a day and the guidelines for mature or aging skin should be followed. After cleansing, splash the face with cool water and pat dry.

Toning: Use a toner designed for normal skin and apply it on the face and neck, using a cotton ball. Leave the skin slightly damp.

Moisturizing: Apply a light moisturizer, or facial oil only where it is needed—usually in the cheek area.

Special Treatments for Normal Skin

Steaming is good for normal skin—once a week for eight to ten minutes.

Exfoliate on a daily basis with an alpha hydroxy acid or papaya enzyme product. Exfoliation will help maintain normal skin and is a good prevention measure against the build-up of dead skin cells that can cause roughness, fine lines, and wrinkles.

Aromatherapy treatments such as facial oils, misters, moisturizers or masks can help to maintain the balance of normal skin. Those containing essential oils of lavender, jasmine, ylang ylang, rosewood, clary sage, and geranium are good choices.

Clay masks, used twice a month, help to deep-clean normal skin. Cream masks may also be used if soothing and nourishing are needed.

Eye creams help prevent the visible signs of aging around the eyes. As time passes, this will be the first place that normal skin develops wrinkles. Using a lightweight moisturizer or specially designed eye cream will protect this area.

Misting is good for normal skin to maintain hydration and is an excellent preventive measure against dryness and wrinkling.

A Suggested Routine For Normal Skin

Daily: *In the morning:* Compress, cleanse, tone, apply an oil-free alpha hydroxy acid product, and moisturize where necessary. Apply lip balm. Mist.

In the evening: Compress, cleanse, tone, and apply an aromatherapy facial skin oil designed for normal skin. Apply an eye cream or light moisturizer around the eyes. Apply lip balm. Mist.

Weekly: Use a papaya enzyme mask.

Steam for eight to ten minutes.

Use a cream mask if the skin needs hydrating and nourishing; use a clay mask if the skin needs a deep cleansing.

Oily Skin

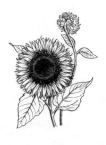

Characteristics: *medium to large pores, shiny appearance, tendency for blackheads and blemishes*

The program for oily skin is designed to keep the skin *well-cleansed without causing dryness* and, because oily skin is prone to blemishes, to *prevent "breakouts."* See Part II to learn how to benefit oily skin using alternative techniques.

The Steps for Oily Skin

Compressing: Use cool to slightly warm compresses. Cool water helps to sedate the oil glands and calm down oil production. (For more information, see Chapter 3, "Skin Care Treatments," under "Compressing.")

Cleansing: In the process of trying to keep oily skin from feeling oily or greasy, it is a common mistake to over-cleanse, causing oily skin to become dehydrated. It can also stimulate oil production as the skin tries to replace the oil that is constantly being cleansed away. Those with oily skin need to resist the temptation to over cleanse by using too harsh a cleanser, to cleanse too often, or to cleanse too vigorously.

Oily skin should to be gently cleansed twice a day— in the morning and before going to bed. Those with younger oily skin should use a cleansing gel or soap-free foaming cleanser that rinses away easily and thoroughly and should avoid any cleansers that contain oil. For maturing oily skin, a milky cleanser can be used, as long as the cleanser is well formulated and rinses well. Oily skin at any age should avoid heavy cream cleansers. Following cleansing, splash the face well with cool water.

Toning: Use a toner designed for oily skin. Be certain that it is alcohol-free. Some manufacturers put alcohol in toners for oily skin but alcohol is too drying for all skin types.

Moisturizing: Younger oily skin will probably not need a moisturizer at all, unless it is dehydrated (lacking water). In this case, use an oil-free moisturizer and only on the areas that need it such as around the eyes and on the cheeks. Facial oils are not recommended because they contain oil, unnecessary for this skin type, and they do not contain water, an ingredient that many oily skins *do* need. Older oily skin will probably be dehydrated and will benefit from the protective and hydrating qualities of a moisturizer. Even for adult oily skin, the moisturizer should be oil-free. However, well-formulated light creams or lotions can be used.

Special Treatments for Oily Skin

Steaming helps to deep-clean oily skin. Once or twice a week for eight to ten minutes is good. Steaming helps keep the pores clear and prevents clogging that may lead to blackheads or blemishes.

Exfoliate using an oil-free alpha hydroxy acid product. This will also help keep the pores clean and un-clogged, which helps prevent blemishes.

Aromatherapy treatments can be very beneficial for oily skin to help balance glandular activity, improve circulation, and detoxify. Look for products such as masks, toners and misters, that contain essential oils of lavender, geranium, ylang ylang, peppermint, juniper (berry), orange, cypress, lemon, clary sage, or tea tree.

Clay masks are well suited for oily skin for deep cleansing and detoxifying. Cream masks should not be used.

Because the eye area produces almost no oil for protection, even those with oily skin should be using an **eye cream** in a light formulation.

Facial misting is good for oily skin to help maintain the moisture balance.

A Suggested Routine For Oily Skin

Daily: *In the morning:* Compress, cleanse, tone, and apply an oil-free alpha hydroxy acid product. If the skin is dehydrated apply a very light oil-free moisturizer, only where needed. Apply lip balm. Mist.

During the day, if necessary: Wipe the face with a cotton ball saturated with a toner or aloe vera juice.

Evening: Compress, cleanse, and tone. Use a hydrating, light moisturizer or eye cream around the eyes. Mist.

Once or Twice Weekly: Steam for eight to ten minutes.

Use a clay-based mask.

Special Considerations for Oily Skin

1. Dietary considerations: Raw and steamed fruits and vegetables have a cleansing, non-congesting effect on oily skin. Animal fats and dairy products can aggravate an oily skin condition. In addition to the vitamins and minerals important for skin health, lecithin can be taken as a supplement and may benefit oily skin by helping to emulsify the oils in the body, helping to prevent skin congestion and clogged pores. (For more information, See Chapter 16, "Nutrition.")

2. Stress can stimulate oil production in the skin by affecting the hormone levels in the bloodstream.

3. Whenever you have spent a lot of times outdoors or driving on the freeway, wipe your face with a cotton pad dampened with a non-drying toner or aloe vera. Pollutants and dirt in the air will adhere to oily skin and can cause blemish problems.

4. Do not use soap on oily skin. It is too drying and irritating, which can stimulate oil production. Soap residue does not rinse well from the skin and can also block pores and cause blemishes.

5. Avoid frequent facial massage because it can stimulate oil production.

6. Avoid products that contain alcohol. Alcohol aggravates oily skin and dries it out. Prolonged use of alcohol-based products causes dehydration, pore enlargement, and a leathery texture.

7. Too little sleep and chronic fatigue can aggravate an oily skin condition.

Dry Skin

Characteristics: *a tight feel to the skin, dull appearance, fine texture, may have visible flaking*

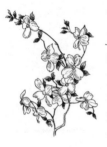

The skin care program for dry skin is designed to *protect the skin from moisture loss* and *prevent damage* from harsh conditions such as wind, extreme temperatures, and sun exposure. This is accomplished by using the right cosmetics and techniques to prevent further drying and by keeping the skin well hydrated both internally and externally. See Part II to learn how to benefit dry skin using alternative techniques.

The Steps for Dry Skin

Compressing: Dry skin—whether lacking oil, water, or both—will greatly benefit from plenty of warm facial compresses because they stimulate glandular function and hydrate the skin. Avoid cold water or prolonged cool-water rinsing because it slows down the sebaceous glands and oil production, which is not good for dry skin. (For more information, see Chapter 3, "Skin Care Treatments," under "Compressing.")

Cleansing: Cleansing *one time a day* is all that is necessary for dry skin, and this is best done in the evening. Milky cleansers are best for dry skin although creamy cleansers can also be used. In the morning, splash the face with warm water or use warm facial compresses. Pat dry excess moisture but leave the skin slightly damp and then apply your moisturizer. NEVER use soap on

	dry skin and avoid abrasive scrubs. "Deep pore" cleansers are not necessary for dry skin, as the pores are often very small and dirt and debris tend to sit on the surface of the skin.
Toning:	Be certain that your toner is formulated for dry skin and does not contain any ingredients that could cause further dryness or irritation. This includes alcohol, artificial colors, and artificial fragrances. Toning is optional for dry skin. If you feel that you are able to thoroughly rinse the cleanser from the skin, you may choose not to use a toner.
Moisturizing:	For regular use, dry skin needs a medium to heavy, well-balanced moisturizer with a very good humectant. If dry skin is exposed to cold or wind or dry air, a heavier moisturizer should be used to provide increased protection. Avoid the tendency to suffocate dry skin with heavy creams all of the time. Overuse of heavy moisturizers will discourage the natural production of oil.

Facial oils are not recommended for dry skin as a moisturizer because they do not contain water in the formulation, an ingredient that dry skin desperately needs, however, they can be used as nutritive treatments.

Special Treatments for Dry Skin

Frequent **steaming** is not appropriate for dry skin. However, dry skin can steam once or twice a month for the hydrating benefits. Steam at a distance from the skin for two to five minutes. No heat should be felt.

Exfoliation is important for dry skin, especially because it is only cleansed once a day. But because dry skin can also be delicate, use exfoliants carefully. The papaya enzyme exfoliating products are gentle enough for dry skin. The alpha hydroxy acid products may also work well, but use them carefully and if there is any sign of irritation, reduce the frequency of use or discontinue use.

Aromatherapy treatments are good for dry skin if they provide moisture and oil as well as the essential oils such as a moisturizer or a cleansing milk. The essential oils that benefit dry skin include lavender, sandalwood, and geranium because they help to balance the glandular function in the skin. The gentle essential oils such as rose, neroli, and chamomile (Roman) are good for dry skin that is irritated or delicate.

Hydrating masks are excellent for dry skin and can be used once a week, or more often, if necessary. Do not use clay-based masks unless they contain ingredients that counteract the drying effects of clay.

Eye creams are very important and should be worn during the day and at night. The eye cream should be a gentle formulation that contains good humectants, water and oils.

Misting may be the single best treatment for dry skin—as long as it is done while wearing a moisturizer with a good humectant. Mist throughout the day and as often as possible.

A Suggested Routine For Dry Skin

Daily: *In the morning:* Splash the face with warm water. Use an alpha hydroxy acid product for exfoliation, if your skin can tolerate it. Apply a moisturizer with a good humectant such as glycerin, panthenol, or hyaluronic acid on the entire face. Apply an eye cream and a lip balm. Mist.
Evening: Compress, cleanse, tone (optional), and moisturize with an aromatherapy skin cream or lotion. Apply an eye cream and a lip balm. Mist. Do not sleep with a heavy night cream.

Weekly: Use a hydrating and/or conditioning cream mask. If you are unable to use an alpha hydroxy acid product, use a papaya enzyme mask once a week. In this case, you would be using a mask twice a week—once for exfoliating and once for hydrating. Begin with the enzyme mask, then in two or three days use the cream mask.

Monthly: Steam, as described under "Special Treatments" above, once or twice a month.

Special Considerations for Dry Skin

1. Dry skin can be caused and aggravated by frequent swimming in chlorinated pools and frequent exposure to wind and salt water.

If you swim often, rinse the skin well *every time* you get out of the water. If you are often exposed to wind and salt water, wear a heavy moisturizer for protection.

2. Some acne medications can cause severe surface dryness. If you have blemish problems, you probably are not a dry skin type. See recommendations for Oily or Blemished Skin and follow the suggested guidelines.

3. Air travel in pressurized cabins dehydrates the skin. If you fly frequently, drink plenty of water and mist your face often while wearing a moisturizer that contains a good humectant.

4. Overconsumption of alcohol will contribute to dehydration of the skin.

5. Be aware that dieting can create a dry skin condition if oils have been eliminated from the diet. The body *needs* a certain amount of oil every day to provide the essential fatty acids that are necessary both for healthy skin and a healthy body. Oils should not be eliminated from the diet for a long period of time. If this is necessary, essential fatty acids should be supplemented.

6. Harsh cosmetics can cause/aggravate dry skin.

7. Dry skin can benefit from nutritional supplementation. Vitamin A keeps the skin supple and relieves roughness. The B vitamins help to balance the skin's glandular activity. Vitamin C assists glandular activity and is also crucial to the formation of collagen and elastin, the building blocks of the skin. Vitamin E softens skin and is required for tissue metabolism. It also conserves oxygen, slowing the signs of aging. Essential fatty acids help to keep the skin youthful.

8. Drinking plenty of water is important for dry skin as an *internal* moisturizer.

9. Avoid diuretic foods such as coffee, tea, cranberry juice, parsley, watercress, spinach, and eggplant because they cause the body to lose water.

10. If you have truly dry skin yet the pores are dilated, it may be the result of using creams which are too rich, left on too long, or used in too great a quantity.

11. Avoid cold water on the face. It slows and suppresses the glandular activity and circulation, both of which need to be stimulated, not suppressed, in dry skin.

12. Overusing powder cosmetics such as blushers and translucent powders can be drying to the skin.

13. Always protect dry skin from sun damage with a sunblock.

14. Try not to let your shampoo run down over your face when you rinse your hair. Shampoos are made with detergents and are far too strong for the facial skin.

15. Keep all hair products off the facial skin, especially hair spray—it can be drying as well as irritating.

16. Use humidifiers in rooms that are artificially heated to replace the moisture in the air that is lost to the dry heat.

Combination Skin

Characteristics: *two or more distinctly different areas on the face*

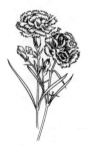

The skin care program for combination skin is designed to help *balance* the separate areas of skin with distinctly different characteristics. Almost every skin type has a slightly more oily "T" zone which includes the forehead, nose, and sometimes the chin. The cheeks and the area around the eyes are usually drier. So, unless the difference between these two areas is extreme, the skin does not need to be treated as if it were two skins, needing two separate sets of products. An example of combination skin with an extreme difference is one with a very oily, perhaps blemished, nose and forehead combined with dry, maybe chapped and flaky skin on the cheeks. When this is the case, the two areas need to be treated as two separate skins—trying to benefit each area and to encourage a state of balance.

The Steps for Combination Skin

Compressing: Warm compresses work well for combination skin. If the areas are extreme, follow the guidelines given for each type in their separate sections of this chapter. (For more information, see Chapter 3, "Skin Care Treatments," under "Compressing".)

Cleansing: Combination skin should be cleansed twice a day—morning and evening—if the skin is mostly normal/oily. If the skin is mostly normal/dry, then cleanse only once a day. If the degree of difference between the areas is slight, then you should be able to use the same cleanser for the whole face. If you are using only one cleanser, it should be is designed for the least oily area. It is better for your complexion to under-clean the oily part than to over-clean the drier part. If the degree of difference is extreme, each area will need to be cleansed with a product designed for that type of skin. Follow the guidelines given for each type in their separate sections of this chapter.

Toning: Use the same guidelines for the toner as the cleanser: depending on the degree of difference in the two areas of skin, you may need to use two different formulas. Or, you may use a toner on the oilier area of the skin and none on the drier part.

Moisturizing: A moisturizer should be used on the drier areas of combination skin, and use your discretion on the oily areas. If the oily areas are dehydrated, use an oil-free moisturizer. Follow the guidelines given for each type in their separate sections of this chapter.

Special Treatments for Combination Skin

For combination skin that is not extreme and has normal/dry characteristics, follow the Special Treatments guidelines for dry skin. If it has normal/oily characteristics, refer to the Special Treatments section for normal skin. If the areas are extreme, treat each area individually, following the guidelines given for each type of skin in the separate sections of this chapter. See Part II to learn how to benefit combination skin using alternative techniques.

A Suggested Routine for Combination Skin

If the skin's differences are extreme, for the daily (morning and evening), weekly, and monthly routine, follow the guidelines for each skin type as described in the separate sections of this chapter. If the skin is not extreme and has normal/dry characteristics, treat the total skin as if it were dry (see "A Suggested Routine for Dry Skin"). If the skin is not extreme and has normal/oily characteristics, treat the total skin as if it were normal (see "A Suggested Routine for Normal Skin").

Special Considerations for Combination Skin

To understand the special considerations for each area of combination skin, refer to the section for that skin type in this chapter. For example, if you have dry skin in one area, refer to the section on "Dry Skin." If your skin is oily in one area, refer to the section on "Oily Skin."

Sensitive Skin

*Characteristics: delicate; over-reacts to sun,
touch, and certain cosmetic ingredients*

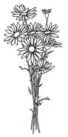

Sensitive skin needs special, gentle care. Each case must receive individual attention because sensitivities can vary. The skin care program for sensitive skin is designed to *calm the skin* and *prevent irritation* by using simple, gentle techniques; by using and varying products that are well-tolerated; and by eliminating the conditions that cause problems. It may be necessary to try several different brands of skin care products to find one that works effectively without irritating. Be certain to read product ingredient labels and avoid artificial colors and fragrances— they are known irritants that frequently cause allergic reactions.

If you have sensitive skin, pay close attention to it. If it becomes irritated from any part of your skin care program such as the type of cleanser, the temperature of the water, the number of times you cleanse, the toner, or the moisturizer—the program will need to be changed. Certain parts may need to be eliminated. Many sensitive-skinned people make their own cosmetics so they can completely avoid the ingredients they know they are allergic to. Remember: the simpler, the better for sensitive skin—both in product ingredients and routine. See Part II to learn how to benefit sensitive skin using alternative techniques.

The Steps for Sensitive Skin

Compressing: Use tepid or warm facial compresses, not hot or cold. (For more information, see Chapter 3, "Skin Care Treatments," under "Compressing.")

Cleansing: Sensitive skin should only be cleansed one time a day—in the evening—using a milky or creamy cleanser. NEVER use soap on sensitive skin and never use scrubs or abrasive cleansers. Avoid cleansers with complicated and elaborate ingredients. Again, the simpler the better—as long as the ingredients are safe and natural. When using the cleanser, press, pat, and smooth it gently over the face. Do not rub!

Toning: Toning is optional for sensitive skin. If you choose not to use a toner, you must be certain that you thoroughly rinse the cleanser from your skin. If residue from the cleanser is left on the skin, it could be irritating. If you do use a toner, use it sparingly, and only if your skin can tolerate it. It may be necessary to dilute the toner with water to make it more gentle.

Moisturizing: Sensitive skin needs a good protective barrier because it can be irritated and damaged by extreme temperatures, pollution, and other environmental conditions. Just like other products for sensitive skin, the moisturizer should be simply formulated, without artificial colors or fragrances. Some active ingredients such as essential oils, may be too active for very sensitive skin. Facial oils can be used if the skin is not dehydrated.

Special Treatments for Sensitive Skin

If sensitive skin is **steamed,** the source of steam should be a distance from the face so that it is not hot on the skin. This distance will need to be determined at the time you are steaming. For some steamers your face will be a foot away, for others it may only be six inches—but you should not feel any *heat* from the steam on your face. Steam for only two to three minutes and only once or twice a month. Then, decide whether or not your skin is profiting from regular steaming. It may not be a necessary or beneficial part of sensitive skin care.

Exfoliation is not generally recommended for sensitive skin because it can be irritating. Yet, exfoliation may be beneficial and, in some cases, it is well tolerated, depending on the sensitivities of the skin. Of the two most popular exfoliants, green papaya and alpha hydroxy acids, the green papaya is better suited for sensitive skin.

Sensitive skin can benefit from the rejuvenating and nourishing qualities of essential oils and **aromatherapy treatments** but some very sensitive skins cannot tolerate them. Look for products such as moisturizers, misters, and cleansers that contain very gentle essential oils such as chamomile (Roman), lavender, and rose in a low percentage such as 1 percent.

Both clay-based **masks** and cream masks may be used by sensitive skin, depending on the ingredients and the level of skin sensitivity. If the skin is dry and sensitive, use cream masks. If the skin is oily and sensitive, clay masks may be beneficial. Clay, in itself, is not a known allergen. If you choose to use a cream mask, check the ingredients. It may be wise for sensitive-skinned people to make their own masks. (See Chapter 7, "Making Your Own Skin Care Products.")

Eye creams are helpful for sensitive skin to protect the delicate eye area. As always, carefully check the ingredients for items you cannot tolerate.

Misting is a wonderfully refreshing and hydrating skin care treatment and it is usually well tolerated by sensitive skin. For skin that is irritated or inflamed, misting the face with chamomile tea can be very soothing.

A Suggested Routine for Sensitive Skin

Daily: *In the morning:* Because sensitive skin requires only one thorough cleansing a day, just splash your face with warm water or use warm-water compresses. Apply a moisturizer, an eye cream, and lip balm. Mist.
  In the evening: Compress, cleanse, tone (optional), and moisturize with a light moisturizer, a small amount of jojoba oil, or a gentle aromatherapy facial oil. Apply an eye cream and lip balm. Mist.

Weekly: Use a papaya enzyme exfoliating mask, if your skin can tolerate it.

Monthly: Steam once or twice a month if you have decided it is helpful for your skin.

Special Considerations for Sensitive Skin

1. The most common place for sensitive skin to react to cosmetics is next to the nose and on the eyelids.

2. As many as one in four people react negatively to artificial fragrances in products.[1]

3. If you are extremely sensitive and hesitate to try new products (or to use *any* product) because you do not want to risk a reaction on your face, do a patch test first. Apply a small amount of the product on your inner elbow or behind your ear and cover with a small gauze pad or bandage. Leave in place, undisturbed, for 24 hours. Usually, any sensitive reaction will occur in that time. If there is no reaction, the product should be safe to use.

4. When trying new products in your skin care program, introduce only one at a time. In this way, if you have a reaction, you will know exactly which product caused it.

5. Sensitive skin has a tendency to develop allergic reactions (sensitivities) to products that are used all the time. It is wise to rotate or change any products used on a regular basis. This is especially important for products that are left on the skin such as moisturizers.

6. Be aware that a product labeled "hypoallergenic" is not a guarantee that you will not have an allergic reaction. "Hypoallergenic" means that in testing, *fewer* people reacted to the ingredients.

7. Not everyone who thinks they have sensitive skin actually does. Even "normal" skin may exhibit signs of sensitivity when it is over-cleansed, damaged by the sun, or exposed to extreme weather conditions.

8. To help calm sensitive skin that is red or irritated: Try cool water compresses, calamine lotion, or chamomile tea compresses.

Blemished Skin

Characteristics: *chronic blemishes,
whiteheads, or blackheads; overactive oil glands*

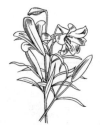

The skin care program for blemished skin is designed to *find the imbalance* that causes the blemishes and to compensate by making changes in diet, life style, and skin care habits. The gentle, external skin care program is designed to *calm and purify* the skin.

There is no medical cure for the cause of blemishes, though the symptoms can be treated with drugs such as antibiotics and Accutane. Finding one cure for blemishes is not possible because of the biochemical and physiological differences that cause the problem in individual acne sufferers—so, there is no single solution that will work for everyone. Approaching and eliminating the cause of blemished skin with natural methods requires time and a process of trial and error. A significant difference may take as long as three months to achieve. However, when the answer has been found, it can be a permanent answer and not just a temporary solution, which is a drawback to drug therapy.

The Steps for Blemished Skin

Compressing: Use cool to slightly warm facial compresses. (For more information, see Chapter 3, "Skin Care Treatments," under "Compressing.")

Cleansing: Blemished skin should be cleansed well, two times a day, morning and evening. Do not use a cream cleanser and *do not over cleanse* with a strong, drying cleanser. In particular, do not use soap because it can irritate the skin and clog the pores, causing more blemishes. Cleansing gels are well suited for younger blemished skin. Gels and some well-formulated cleansing milks can be used for adult blemished skin. Whatever cleanser is chosen, it must rinse easily and thoroughly from the skin.

Toning: Use a toner made especially for blemished skin. Aloe vera and herbal extract-based toners can be excellent for blemished skin, if well formulated. Look for ingredients that calm and purify such as chamomile, lavender, juniper, and sage.

Moisturizing: Moisturizers may not be necessary unless the skin is dehydrated. In this case, use only an oil-free moisturizer. Facial oils are not recommended for blemished skin.

Special Treatments for Blemished Skin

Steaming helps to cleanse by encouraging perspiration, cleansing the pores from the inside out and allowing the oil to flow freely. Steaming can be used as often as twice a week for eight to ten minutes if it has been determined to be helpful. Because blemished skin needs to be treated gently, be certain not to "burn" the skin with steam by having the steam source too close to the skin. The steam should feel warm and gentle, not hot.

Exfoliation is often helpful for blemished skin. Alpha hydroxy acid products can prevent the pores from clogging with cellular debris. This can help prevent blemishes. Choose an oil-free, liquid product. Watch for skin irritation. If this occurs, use a milder AHA product or use it less often. Never use abrasive scrubs or sponges on blemished skin.

Aromatherapy treatments can be very effective for helping blemished skin. All essential oils have antibacterial properties and are easily absorbed into the skin to serve this purpose. Choose aromatherapy products such as misters, toners and oil-free moisturizers. Lavender and geranium are excellent to help balance oil production and fight bacteria. Juniper (berry) is an excellent detoxifier, and tea tree oil helps the immune system. Chamomile (Roman) is a superb anti-inflammatory.

Clay masks are very good for blemished skin because they help to absorb oil and toxins. Do not use cream masks.

Eye creams are important for all skin types, including blemished skin. The eye area has very few oil glands and is not a blemish-prone area. Use a lightweight eye cream, sparingly, as a protectant.

Misting is well-suited for blemished skin, as this type of skin still needs moisture. It can be helpful to add essential oils to the misting water or to use an herb tea. (See Chapter, "Making Your Own Skin Care Products.")

A Suggested Routine for Blemished Skin

Daily: *In the morning:* Compress, cleanse, tone, apply an alpha hydroxy acid product that is oil-free, moisturize if necessary with an oil-free moisturizer. Apply a light eye cream and a lip balm. Mist.

At mid-day: Some people with blemishes feel it is beneficial to do a mini-cleansing treatment during the day. This can be done with compresses, cool-water splashes, or a clean cotton pad dampened with toner or aloe vera juice.

In the evening: Compress, cleanse, tone, and apply an oil-free moisturizer, if the skin feels dehydrated. Apply eye cream and lip balm. Mist.

Weekly: Steam the face once or twice a week for eight to ten minutes and then follow with a clay-based mask. Be certain that the clay is rinsed thoroughly from the skin, otherwise it may clog the pores and be irritating.

Special Considerations for Blemished Skin

1. The sun can be used therapeutically for blemished skin but only in very small doses. Too much sun will aggravate oil production and can cause surface burning, which will trap oils underneath the top layer of skin, possibly causing blemishes to worsen.

2. Never squeeze a blemish in the "triangle of death." This is the area from the corners of the lips to the bridge of the nose. It is possible for the infection to spread into the sinus cavity, which has been known to be fatal.

3. People with a history of taking antibiotics can develop acne because of the disruption of the "good" and "bad" bacteria in the intestines. This disruption can be alleviated by taking an acidophilus supplement and minimizing sweet foods to help re-establish the beneficial intestinal flora. Prolonged antibiotic use should be avoided, if possible.

4. Constipation can cause skin breakouts. Increasing dietary fiber and water intake can help relieve constipation.

5. Stress can stimulate hormone and glandular function, thereby increasing oil production, which can aggravate an acne condition. Practice helpful stress-reduction techniques. (See Chapter 19, "Managing Stress.")

6. Oriental medicine maintains that the area of the face where blemishes have appeared is a clue to internal imbalances. Blemishes on the forehead can indicate a problem in the intestinal area. Blemishes on the cheeks indicate the lungs and around the mouth is the reproductive area. Between the eyebrows is the liver, and the shoulders indicate the digestive system.

7. Remember that chronic blemishes are not just a skin problem. They are a symptom of a systemic/internal imbalance that is reflected on the skin. Blemished skin is influenced by age (especially puberty, when hormonal changes affect the oil glands), diet, poor elimination, allergies, cosmetics, certain medications, disease, heredity, and/or stress. Acne must be approached with internal considerations such as diet, vitamins, and exercise, as well as external care. Using just an external skin care program will not solve the problem of blemished skin.

8. Do not use abrasive sponges or granular cleansers. These can be irritating and can spread an infection.

9. Smoking aggravates a blemished condition because it restricts the circulation of vital nutrients to the skin and slows the healing process.

10. The skin is only one of the eliminative organs of the body. Other eliminative organs include the lungs, the liver, the kidneys, and the intestines.

Eliminating blemishes may require that all of the eliminative organs are working at their best.

11. Blemished skin should not be covered with make-up on a regular basis because it can make the condition worse. This is especially true for poorly formulated products with ingredients that may irritate the skin and clog the pores. If it is absolutely necessary, wear make-up over blemished skin only on special occasions and then clean it off as soon as possible.

12. Blemished skin should not be vigorously massaged. This can stimulate oil production and result in further clogging of the pores. It can also spread infection.

13. Sunscreens have been known to promote or aggravate blemishes. If you have blemished skin and regularly use a sunscreen, stop using it for a period of time to see if the blemished condition improves.

14. Hair products such as mousse, gel, or spray can cause blemishes, especially under bangs and around the hairline.

15. Certain toothpastes, especially tartar-control, can cause blemishes around the mouth.

Alternative Techniques for Blemished Skin

1. **Castor Oil** is an exceptional healing medium used for inflammation, swellings, and bruises. Castor oil is from the seed of the castor oil plant, also known as the Palma Christi (Palm of Christ). It is claimed to have wonderful healing powers when applied to the skin. Its action is nutritive, soothing, and cleansing.

Though castor oil can be applied (sparingly) directly to the affected areas, it is best used on the abdomen/stomach in the form of a pack (a piece of folded white flannel, saturated with castor oil), covered with plastic and then warmed with either a hot water bottle or an electric heating pad. (Certain conditions such as appendicitis or other acute infections require that the oil *not* be heated.) The castor pack's physiological effects include improved elimination, assimilation, lymphatic circulation, and the drawing out of infection. The pack applied to the abdomen/stomach area is effective regardless of the location of the inflammation in the body. Constituents of the oil are absorbed through the skin and walls of the small intestine, where they aid the lymphatic system to keep the body free of toxins. The beneficial effects are then transmitted through the intestinal tract to the internal organs to stimulate healing and break up congestion.

For chronic blemishes, try the castor oil skin pack three times in one week for one and a half hours each time. This series can be repeated if necessary and may be used on a maintenance basis, either monthly or bi-monthly. The castor pack can be stored in the refrigerator and used twenty times before needing to replace the oil and clean the cloth.

2.   **Homeopathic** remedies are available for blemished skin and many natural food stores carry them. Silica 6c is recommended for scarring acne where pimples are slow to change; hepar sulph 6c for large, infected pimples that discharge; and belladonna 6c for red, inflamed pimples. The remedy should be taken once a day for no longer than a month. If the remedy is going to work for you, you will see results in two weeks. Though these remedies can be used with no background knowledge about homeopathy, results are often more effective and long-lasting when the medicine is prescribed by an experienced homeopathic doctor. An excellent introductory book to this 200-year-old system of healing is *Everybody's Guide to Homeopathic Medicine,* by Stephen Cummings and Dana Ullman (see Bibliography).

3.   The **Aromatherapy** essential oils used for blemished skin are listed below.
Cedarwood is valuable in all types of skin eruptions because of its sedative, astringent and antiseptic qualities. It helps to balance oil production.
Chamomile (Roman) is soothing and reduces inflammation, dryness, itching, and redness.
Clary Sage relieves inflammation, and promotes cell regeneration. It helps to control excessive oil production.
Frankincense is anti-bacterial and soothing. It helps to balance oil production and stimulates cellular renewal.
Geranium reduces inflammation and helps to balance glandular activity. It stimulates circulation and the regeneration of skin cells.

Helichrysum stimulates the production of new cells, and reduces inflammation.
Juniper (berry) stimulates circulation and purifies the blood. It is an excellent cleanser, astringent and antiseptic. It also encourages perspiration which is cleansing for blemished skin. It helps to balance oil production.
Lavender soothes and reduces inflammation, while helping to balance glandular activity. It is also an excellent antiseptic.
Rosewood encourages cell rejuvenation, is soothing, and helps to balance oil production.
Sandalwood has emollient and sedative qualities and is very good for chronic inflammations. It helps to balance oil production.
Tea tree is a powerful antiseptic and supports the immune system.
Ylang ylang helps to balance oil production, fights bacterial infection, and stimulates new cell growth.

4. **Bach Flower Remedies** were created by Dr. Edward Bach, a British bacteriologist and homeopath who left a lucrative practice in the 1930's to devote the last six years of his life to search for a simple, natural method of healing. He believed that emotional and psychological difficulties such as worry, loneliness, sadness, and fear open the pathway to the invasion of illness, reduce our resistance to disease, as well as prevent the healing process. He believed if his patients were in a balanced emotional state, this would assist, if not induce, a return to good health and that there was no true healing unless there was a change in attitude that brought peace of mind and inner happiness.

As a result of this search, Dr. Bach developed the Bach Flower Remedies, thirty-eight flower essences designed to relieve mental distress. They are made from blossoms and buds. When these remedies are taken orally, they act as catalysts to revitalize and awaken one's innate ability to balance and heal. Their action is very gentle and strengthening. They are non-toxic and non-addictive and have been successful not only with children and adults but also plants and animals. They do not have a specific pharmacological effect on the body; rather, they assist in realigning the subtle electromagnetic field that surrounds the body and each cell. In doing this, the Bach Flower Remedies use the plant's properties to harmonize, balance, and stabilize emotional sensitivities.

Jane Bell, a certified Flower Essence counselor, is a devoted and skilled prac-
titioner of this healing art. Jane notes that blemished skin will often have underlying emotional causes that can be addressed by the Bach Flower Remedies. She
says that in selecting the appropriate remedy, one looks at the personality of the
individual rather than the problem itself.[2] Following are a few possible scenarios
to help people with blemished skin discern the corresponding remedies.

a. For those who are easily discouraged over minor setbacks, or who cry or
    give up easily—use Gentian.

b. For those who feel life is unfair and that they are being "picked on"—
    use Willow.

c. For those who are hostile, jealous, vengeful, or rebellious—use Holly.

d. For those who lose their self-confidence or feel like "I can't do it"—
    use Larch.

e. For those who are weak-willed, anxious to please, and easily exploited—
    use Centaury.

f. For those who are experiencing emotional upsets due to transition and
    change (such as puberty)—use Walnut.

g. For those who are obsessed with bodily impurities and imperfection—
    use Crab Apple.

h. For those who are very self-critical and get stuck in self-blame—use Pine.

I. For those who are tense, impatient or irritated—use Impatiens.

j. For those who feel overwhelmed by their duties and responsibilities—
    use Elm.

k. Rescue Remedy, a unique combination of flower essences designed by
    Bach, is suggested for flare-ups of blemishes. Rescue Remedy can be put
    directly on the blemishes as well as in a glass of water (three drops) and
    sipped throughout the day.

For Recommended Reading about Bach Flower Remedies, see Chapter 19,
"Managing Stress."

5. **Allergy Testing** for unknown food allergies can be one of the most singu-
larly successful approaches to chronic blemishes. It requires a very specific
method of testing, using a blood sample. This testing is done by ImmunoLabs in

Florida (800-231-9197) and at Immuno Diagonostic Labs in California (707-765-6586). It is not necessary to travel to these locations to be tested. The test reveals the foods to which you are allergic and the degree of the allergic reaction. By eliminating the offending foods from your diet, a number of physical complaints such as fatigue, headaches, nausea, arthritis, digestive problems, and blemishes can be relieved.

6.   An **Ayurvedic** approach holds that blemishes represent an imbalanced condition in the blood and muscle tissue system. To stop blemishes, all the eliminative systems in the body must be working well. This includes the kidneys, liver, lungs, and intestines as well as the skin. All "heating foods" such as garlic, chili, and onions are to be avoided, with a bland diet recommended. For cystic type acne, all dairy products, seafood, and citrus must be eliminated. Weekly facial masks are recommended made with graham flour mixed with a few drops of sandalwood oil and enough water to form a paste. Calamine lotion applied at night and rinsed off in the morning is another Ayurvedic remedy commonly used in India with good results. Drinking one-half cup of aloe vera juice two times a day can also help clear the skin.

7.   **Reflexology** can help counteract the imbalances that cause blemished skin by stimulating internal organs and improving their function. Massaging the correlating areas of the hands and feet stimulate the *liver* to store and release vita-

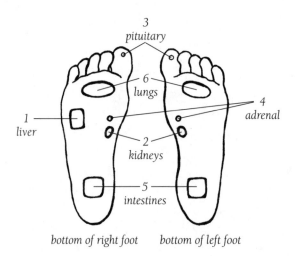

bottom of right foot   bottom of left foot

min A that helps balance the production of skin oil. The liver also helps to regulate nutrient absorption and release antibodies to fight infections. Stimulation of the *kidneys* can help filter toxins from the blood; stimulation of the *pituitary gland* can help to balance the glandular functions and secretion of oil; stimulation of the *adrenal glands* can help fight inflammation of the oil glands; stimulation of the *intestines* can encourage efficient processing of nutrients and regular elimination of waste products; and stimulation of the *lungs* can encourage efficient oxygen supply to the tissues and removal of carbon dioxide.

8.   **Acupressure** can be helpful for the prevention of blemishes by stimulating and toning the complexion and improving overall health. Apply a firm yet gentle pressure to a selected point on the body using the fingertips. The point should be

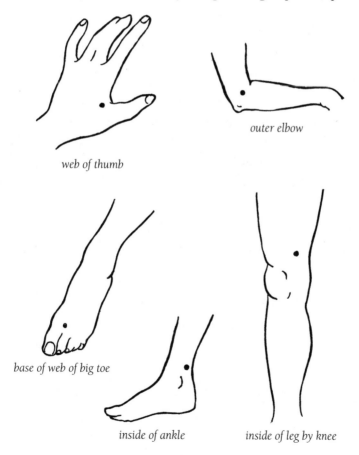

outer elbow

web of thumb

base of web of big toe

inside of ankle   *inside of leg by knee*

pressed for three seconds, released, and then pressed again for three seconds, and so on for thirty counts. These points should be pressed daily and on a regular schedule to be the most effective such as morning, noon, and evening.

Five-Point Stimulation

1. Base of the web of the thumb
2. Outer elbow
3. Base of the web of the big toe
4. Inside of the ankle
5. Inside of the leg by the knee

Together, these points will stimulate detoxification, increase the body's ability to fight infection, reduce stress, and help to balance the hormones. See Chapter 8, "Acupressure," for more details and to learn "Big Washing Face Massage," which is good for blemished skin.

9. **Nutrition** should be the first and foremost consideration for anyone afflicted with chronic blemishes. Annemarie Colbin, author of *Food and Healing* believes that the diet has *everything* to do with blemish problems, including acne. She corrected her own poor skin as well as that of her students afflicted with chronic blemishes within three months of a dietary change. Her primary suggestion is to eliminate dairy products from the diet. Cheese, milk, butter, and ice cream clog the body's filtering systems, especially in people who do not tolerate dairy products well. Eliminating saturated fats, caffeine, and sugar will also help eliminate chronic blemishes.

A diet that promotes a clear complexion is high in fiber and rich in fresh, natural foods, especially steamed and raw vegetables. There must also be enough available protein because amino acids are necessary for the skin to heal and rebuild properly. Be certain to drink plenty of water to flush toxins from the body, and do not overeat because it puts a strain on the systems of the body. Most people respond very well to an improved diet, experiencing a noticeable difference in their skin in one to six months.

After initiating a dietary change, adding vitamin and mineral supplements can be beneficial. Those particularly important for healthy skin are vitamin A to prevent and clear up infections, dryness, and scaliness (try a higher dose than the Recommended Daily Allowance for one month, then drop the dose gradually to the RDA); the vitamin B complex for clear skin, balanced glandular activity, and calm nerves; vitamin C to prevent and clear infections, to strengthen the underlying tissues, and to support cellular repair (2,000 to 5,000 mg vitamin C daily may be helpful); vitamin E to conserve oxygen, help preserve the elasticity of the skin, and accelerate healing; selenium for good skin elasticity; and zinc for the immune system generally, as well as its role in hormone activity and wound healing. Zinc is considered to be the single most important mineral used therapeutically for blemishes and has been known to significantly improve blemishes as well as boils and eczema. Interestingly, the body's need for zinc increases during puberty—the most common time for blemishes. Zinc has antibacterial and anti-inflammatory effects on the skin and also fights free-radical damage.

Other supplements that may prove beneficial are EFAs (essential fatty acids), which are necessary for proper glandular functioning, tissue repair, and immune function. Flax seed oil is an excellent source of EFAs. One tablespoon of flax seed oil is recommended daily. Aloe vera juice can benefit the skin due to its balancing and toning effect on the intestinal tract. Two to four ounces a day consumed internally is recommended. Chlorophyll liquid or tablets and any green foods are very cleansing and healing to the system. If digestion is poor, digestive enzymes such as bromelain, papain, pepsin, or a combination of these may help. Lecithin, either in granular or capsule form, contains B vitamins and helps to emulsify fats and oils in the body. Clay tablets or capsules taken with a large glass of water have a cleansing effect on the intestinal tract and have been successfully used to treat blemished skin. Acidophilus supplements may also be indicated as they restore the beneficial intestinal flora.

Checklist for Blemished Skin

(This is a review of the above information in a format for quick review.)

1. **Diet: Nutrition is the first and foremost consideration for anyone afflicted with chronic blemishes.**
   - ✓ Eliminate dairy products (top priority).
   - ✓ Eliminate saturated fats, sugar, and caffeine.
   - ✓ Increase consumption of fresh, raw, and steamed vegetables and fruit.
   - ✓ Consume adequate amounts of quality protein to heal and rebuild the skin.
   - ✓ Avoid overeating—it taxes the systems in the body.
   - ✓ Consider supplements such as vitamins, minerals, essential fatty acids, aloe vera, chlorophyll, lecithin, and digestive aids.

2. **Lifestyle:**
   - ✓ Investigate effective alternative therapies.
   - ✓ Don't smoke.
   - ✓ Exercise regularly.
   - ✓ Rest and relax so the skin can heal and rejuvenate.
   - ✓ Cut down on drinking alcoholic beverages, or stop altogether.
   - ✓ Manage stress.

3. **Skin care habits:**
   - ✓ Follow a basic skin care program that supports healthy skin and includes both external and internal approaches.
   - ✓ Use the sun therapeutically for blemished skin but only in very small doses.
   - ✓ Use only high quality natural cosmetics that are designed for blemished skin and avoid using soap.
   - ✓ Handle blemished skin gently to avoid irritation and spread of infection.

Mature or Aging Skin

Characteristics: *dryness, decreased elasticity,*
decreased circulation, fine lines and wrinkles

The skin care program for mature or aging skin is designed to *nurture,*
protect, and *rejuvenate.* Though the skin's ability to repair and respond
slows with age, it does not stop. Mature skin can greatly benefit from
proper care, and it is never too late to start to reap the rewards. All of
us will have aging skin as the years go by, and with proper care, we can
have a vibrant complexion and look beautiful at every age. See Part II
to learn how to benefit mature/aging skin using alternative techniques.

The Steps for Mature or Aging Skin

Compressing: Skin loses its moisture content as it ages and the glandular
function slows down, so plenty of warm compresses are needed
to stimulate circulation and hydrate. (For more information, see
Chapter 3, "Skin Care Treatments," under "Compressing.")

Cleansing: Mature/aging skin should be cleansed only one time a day,
preferably in the evening. In the morning, splash the face with
warm water or use warm facial compresses. Pat dry excess
moisture but leave the skin slightly damp for applying your
moisturizer. Milky or creamy cleansers are the best for mature/
aging skin. NEVER, NEVER use soap or abrasive scrubs.

Toning: Toning is optional but if you choose not to use a toner, be
certain that you are able to completely and thoroughly rinse
the cleanser from your skin. If you use a toner, it must be
designed for mature/aging skin.

Moisturizing: Aging skin needs all the benefits a good moisturizer can provide—effective active ingredients such as essential oils, a good
humectant for hydration, anti-oxidant vitamins and herbs to
fight free-radical damage, and oils for barrier protection.
Facial oils are not recommended for dry skin as a moisturizer
because they do not contain water in the formulation.
However, they can be used as nutritive treatments.

Special Treatments for Mature or Aging Skin

Steaming mature/aging skin will cleanse, hydrate and stimulate circulation and can be done once or twice a month. Keep the source of steam a distance from the face so that the steam does not feel hot on the skin, and steam for only two to five minutes.

Exfoliation products such as alpha hydroxy acid and green papaya are very good for mature/aging skin and can help to keep it soft and smooth while diminishing fine line and wrinkles. Care needs to be taken not to overdue exfoliation because it could cause irritation. If this occurs, simply decrease the number of times the product is used or discontinue use for awhile.

Aromatherapy treatments such as moisturizers, masks, and cleansers have a wonderful rejuvenating effect on mature/aging skin. Essential oils such as neroli, lavender, and frankincense are cytophilactic—they stimulate the production of new cells in the basal layer of the skin. Oils such as lavender, ylang ylang and geranium help balance the glandular functions that slow down with age. Carrot seed has a nourishing, rejuvenating effect. Chamomile (Roman) and rose are very good for skin that has developed the visible thread veins known as couperose.

Hydrating and nourishing **masks** are excellent for mature/aging skin. Do not use clay masks unless they have been formulated to counteract the clay's drying effects.

Eye creams are very important to use on a regular basis—both day and night.

Misting is very helpful when it is used in conjunction with a moisturizer that contains a humectant. Misting hydrates the skin, and if used regularly, can reduce superficial dryness and fine lines.

A Suggested Routine For Mature or Aging Skin

Daily: *In the morning:* Splash your face with warm water. Do not cleanse because mature/aging skin only needs to be cleansed once a day—in the evening. Apply an alpha hydroxy acid product. If it is in a liquid, follow with a moisturizer that contains good humectants. If you use an alpha hydroxy acid product in a cream base, you should not need to apply another moisturizer. Apply eye cream and lip balm and then mist. Mist occasionally throughout the day. *In the evening:* Compress with warm water. Cleanse well, rinse thoroughly and tone. Sparingly apply an aromatherapy facial oil then a lightweight moisturizer or use a cream based aromatherapy moisturizer. Apply eye cream and lip balm. Mist.

Weekly: Use a green papaya enzyme mask for additional exfoliation Nourish and hydrate the skin with a cream mask. (Start with the papaya mask to exfoliate dead skin cells. Wait two or three days and then use the nourishing mask.)

Monthly: Steam once or twice a month, at a distance, for only two to five minutes.

Special Considerations for Mature and Aging Skin

During our lifetime, the quality of our skin changes. It passes from the soft and delicate characteristics of baby skin to childhood's smooth, velvety texture and resilient nature. The teenage years are known for blemish problems and in the mid-twenties, our skin is beginning to mature. By our thirties, we may notice it becoming drier with the first signs of wrinkles, and by forty-something—our skin is aging.

As the skin ages, it becomes drier and loses its elasticity. The skin's rejuvenating capacity (cell renewal) slows down, and the oxygen and nutrient supply decreases with a reduction in circulation. The skin loses water content, containing about 7% water compared to 13% for young skin. Protective oil (sebum) production decreases. These changes take place in the dermal layer of the skin. On the surface of the skin, as the cells work their way up from the dermal layer below, cells are thicker and more dense and have decreased ability to retain moisture. The cells are not well lubricated, because of the decreased oil. This gives mature skin its drier appearance. How fast and to what extent this dermal layer changes depends on three things: your age, your heredity, and your lifestyle.

All of the items in Chapter 1, "The Checklist for Beautiful Skin" are important considerations for preventing premature aging of the skin. In fact, if an effective program is put into practice early in life and before the skin begins to show signs of age, many of the signs could be avoided for a long time.

In addition to The Checklist, there are other considerations for mature skin:

1.   Avoid over-manipulation. This refers to heavy scrubbing, heavy facial massage, and over-stretching the skin while applying make-up or skin care products. The facial skin no longer has as much ability to "bounce back." This over-manipulation encourages the skin to wrinkle and sag.

2.   Avoid over-cleansing. This means two things: washing the face more times than is necessary for the particular skin type and/or using too harsh a cleanser. Over-cleansing is not healthful to the function of the skin because it strips away natural oils and disrupts the protective mantle. This can lead to both dryness and irritation, which is particularly damaging to aging skin. The best cleansers for mature or aging skin are milky or creamy cleansers.

3.   Beware of extreme weight loss. Dieting can affect the skin in two ways. First, most dieting programs are low in fats and oils. The skin needs oils to stay soft and supple. Second, as we get older and our skin's elasticity decreases, it is not able to accommodate extreme swings in weight. A great loss of weight can leave skin wrinkled and saggy. If you are dieting, try to lose the weight slowly, and if you must exclude fats and oils, supplement your diet with essential fatty acids in capsule form.

4.   Give special care to the eye area. The delicate skin around the eyes is the first to show signs of aging, and is very sensitive to mistreatment. Here, the skin has few of the oil and sweat glands necessary to keep it conditioned. The skin is also very thin so moisture evaporates easily, leaving the skin dehydrated. The constant movement of the skin around the eyes also contributes to their early wrinkling, especially squinting and smiling. Preventative care and proper skin care habits can delay aging around the eyes.

When applying moisturizers in the eye area, pat or press them in place to avoid stretching the tissue. If you are in the sun, wear sunglasses large enough to cover the entire eye area. The lenses must be the type that block ultraviolet rays. In cold weather and wind, use a heavier moisturizer for protection. Try not to rub your eyes. It stretches the skin and encourages the formation of "bags." When you apply make-up remover in the eye area, use only a small amount and allow it to sit for a few moments to "melt" the make-up for easy removal. Lastly, avoid using common "kleenex"-type tissues around the eyes. They are made of wood bits that can scratch and irritate the skin.

The skin under the eye is thin and delicate, so it shows irritation easily. It will also stretch to accommodate fluid build up. If puffiness in the eye area is present, it may be caused by lack of sleep (fatigue), though it can also be the result of too much sleep. Sinus, thyroid, or kidney problems may show up as under-eye puffiness, as can the overburdening of the liver and bowel. An increase of hormones can contribute to water retention resulting in eye puffiness. Stress, poor elimination, lack of exercise, allergies which irritate the eye membranes, and a diet too high in salt or alcohol are other contributing factors. Under-eye puffiness can also be caused by cosmetics that are too rich or possibly contaminated. Some product may be getting in the eye and causing irritation.

For temporary relief from eye puffiness, try cold cucumber slices or cold water compresses over closed eyes for fifteen minutes, while lying down with the head slightly elevated. In general, sleeping with the head slightly elevated will help to relieve morning eye puffiness. Another helpful treatment: moisten two black tea bags with water. Squeeze out the excess water and put the tea bags in a plastic bag in the refrigerator for an hour. Apply the cold tea bags to closed eyes and lie down for twenty minutes.

5. Provide nutritional supplementation. To combat the dryness and lack of vitality associated with aging skin, the diet must include plenty of fluids (water, juices, herbal teas), oils (essential fatty acids), and anti-oxidants. Anti-oxidants inhibit free-radical damage that contributes to the aging process. Free-radical damage is caused by exposure to sun, smog, and cigarette smoke as well as by the body's normal chemical processes. Some protective anti-oxidant nutrients are vitamins A, C, and E, selenium, bioflavonoids, and beta carotene. Anti-oxidant activity is also available from herbs such as ginkgo biloba, and green tea.

6. Couperose is often found in mature skin, characterized by broken or distended capillaries (small blood vessels) that can be seen through the surface of

the skin. These show as small, red, spider-web-looking veins and are usually more prominent in thin, fair skin.

Couperose is caused when the blood vessels are not elastic enough to handle the flow of blood that is forced through them. This causes them to break or distend. Extremes of heat or cold, alcoholic beverages, hot and spicy foods, caffeine, and sunbathing can all cause and/or aggravate a couperose condition and should be avoided if couperose is present.

Couperose skin should also be handled gently. Do not use abrasive or scrub-type cleansers. Look for skin care products with gentle, calming ingredients. Avoid stimulating masks and steaming.

Bioflavonoids when combined with vitamin C can be helpful in strengthening the capillary walls and can be helpful in preventing couperose. They are available in supplements. Though a couperose condition is very difficult to reverse with natural methods, it is quite possible to prevent further development.

7.   Give special consideration to the lips. As we age and the skin becomes drier, the lips also become drier and prone to chapping. The skin on the lips is very thin and does not have oil glands to provide protection. Sun and cold exposure are the two main culprits for dry, chapped lips. Licking the lips in an attempt to keep them moist will only aggravate the problem. Lips should be protected with a rich lip balm or cream, and if you are in the sun, be certain to wear a lip balm with a sunblock. Drink plenty of water to moisturize the lips from the inside, and if you are experiencing cracked lips, you may be low in B vitamins.

5

Skin Care for the Body

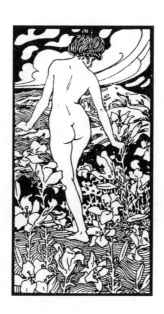

M ost people think of skin care in terms of taking care of the face, but a complete skin care program also includes the body, with special attention for the hands and feet. The natural skin care program for the body is designed to soften, smooth, and rejuvenate and is similar to the care of facial skin but the treatments are slightly different. It includes **cleansing** using either a shower or bath; **stimulating** with dry brush massage or gentle scrubs; **conditioning/nourishing** with custom-made body oils or body packs; **protecting** with body lotion, body oils, or clothing; and **exfoliating** with either mechanical methods or cosmetic exfoliants.

The hands and feet have a special program because they experience more wear and tear than any other part of the body. They also have a unique feature, the nail. Fingernails and toenails can be beautifully groomed with a professional treatment done at home. The hands and feet, pampered with reflexology massage, will not only make them feel wonderful but will benefit the entire body. Special exercises can keep the hands and feet strong and flexible, while observing the guidelines to prevent common problems will keep them in good condition.

5-Part Skin Care for the Body

Cleansing

Cleansing the body removes the excreted wastes and dead skin cells from the surface of the skin, along with accumulated dust and dirt. This can be accomplished by gently scrubbing and then rinsing with water. *The use of soap is not necessary.*

Americans over-cleanse their skin and cause premature aging by using soap too frequently. Cleansing every day with soap is not a custom practiced worldwide. Soap is very harsh and causes the skin to become irritated and dry. It destroys the acid pH mantle on the surface of the skin which was designed to provide protection. It takes time for it to re-establish, once it is removed, and if it is daily washed away, the protection cannot be maintained at its optimum level.

Most of us do not lead the kind of life that necessitates daily bathing, yet this is a common practice. Daily soaping of the entire body or soaking in a tub of soapy water is not good for the skin. Certain areas of the body that have become soiled or perspire heavily, such as under the arms, might be soaped, but the areas that do not need it should be left alone. The shins on the legs, for example, do not have many oil glands, and they will become very dry if soap is used regularly on them. If this concept of not soaping the skin seems unappealing to you, give it a try for two weeks. For your daily bath or shower, simply rinse the skin with water or use a soapless cleanser such as Clay Cleanser listed in Chapter 7, "Making Your Own Skin Care Products." Rinsing is also cleansing but it is not stripping. In the time of two weeks, your skin will feel softer and appear less dry and dull.

For the areas that may require a little soap, choose a glycerin soap (transparent) or a gentle liquid. If you have particularly sensitive or dry skin, dilute one part liquid soap with six parts water. Store it in a squeeze bottle for easy application and use it sparingly. Rinse off all soap very, very well. Remember, *soap is drying and will prematurely age the skin.*

The shower and the bath, America's most common ways to cleanse the body, are actually hydrotherapy (water remedy) treatments, providing the benefits of both the water and the temperature of the water. Warm water has a sedating and relaxing effect, and cool water is refreshing and invigorating. Showers are the more popular in America, probably because they are quick and easy. The bath, however, is gaining popularity because it provides a time for relaxing. The temperature of a bath or shower should always be moderate (about 95-98 degrees). If it is too hot (over 100 degrees) it will encourage couperose, causing veins to appear red and "spidery" on the surface of the skin. It can also drain your energy and dry your skin by removing protective oils. Indeed, a very hot bath can even be dangerous, especially for someone with heart problems. If the temperature is too cold (under 75 degrees), it can depress the body's circulation and also be dangerous, especially after exercising or for people with high blood pressure.

The bath, famous throughout history for its therapeutic and social functions, can be a luxurious and relaxing activity. A warm tub of plain water will not only rinse the skin of the day's soil but will hydrate the skin, relax muscles, and soothe the mind. For a beneficial bathing experience, soak in the tub for about ten to fifteen minutes. If you soak longer, the bath will begin to dry the skin. Avoid putting anything in the bath water that contains soap or artificial ingredients (such as fragrance or color). After bathing, apply a lotion or oil to "seal in" the benefits of the bath's skin hydrating effects. The lotion will help prevent moisture loss.

Following is a list of distinctive baths for you to enjoy that offer the combined benefits of hydrotherapy and special ingredients. It has been said that "baths have as little to do with getting clean as a fine meal has to do with refueling the body's energy supply. A bath, like a good meal, is meant to be savored."[1] Enjoy!

The Aromatherapy Bath

An aromatherapy bath will delightfully pamper and affect you through two of the most powerful sensory organs—the skin and the nose. With the ability of essential oils to lift spirits and relax the body and mind, the bath is an excellent way to experience and enjoy these treasures from nature. Lavender is soothing and promotes a sound sleep. Chamomile (Roman) is calming and relaxing. Both of these are good at the end of the day. Rosemary is stimulating and will clear the mind and is most effective in cooler water—great in the morning! Bergamot is uplifting and has deodorant properties. Marjoram can ease muscular pain and is best used in a warmer bath temperature.

Prepare the essential oil or blend of essential oils for the bath by first diluting it in a carrier base which will help disperse it in the water. (Remember, essential oils and water do not mix. So, essential oils will float on the surface of the water and because they are so concentrated, they could irritate the skin.) Add ten drops of your chosen oils into one tablespoon of vodka or vinegar. Fill the tub with warm water, add the diluted essential oil, and stir well. Immerse yourself and enjoy!

Following are a few suggested aromatherapy baths to try.

The Aromatherapy Cream Bath. Add 5 drops of lavender and 5 drops of chamomile to 1 cup of cream. (The cream will disperse the oils in the water). Pour into a tub of warm water as the tub is filling. This bath is relaxing and very good for dry skin.

The Aromatherapy Wake-up Bath. Blend 5 drops of rosemary, 3 drops of peppermint, and 2 drops of spruce. Add to one tablespoon of vinegar and pour into a tub of water. Stir well. This bath is excellent first thing in the morning.

An Aromatherapy Bath for Hot Days. Blend 5 drops of eucalyptus, 2 drops of peppermint, 2 drops of lemon, and 2 drops of orange. Add to one tablespoon of vinegar and pour into a tub of water. Stir well.

An Aromatherapy Bath for Romance. Blend 5 drops of ylang ylang, 2 drops of sandalwood, 2 drops of lavender and 1 drop of nutmeg. Add to one tablespoon of vinegar and pour into a tub of warm water. Stir well.

The Salt Scrub Bath

For deep pore cleansing, fill the tub with moderate-temperature water and add 2 teaspoons of almond oil. Soak for about 8 minutes then dip your hand into a bowl of sea salt and begin massaging, in circular motions, covering the entire body, except the face. Concentrate on the rougher areas such as the feet, elbows, and knees but **be gentle.** Shower off the salt. This salt scrub bath will leave the skin exceptionally soft and clean.

The Vinegar Bath

Vinegar is an excellent tonic for the skin. It supports the protective acid mantle and can help restore the mantle if it has been removed by chlorine or soap. Vinegar is a soothing cleanser and conditioner. It can ease the discomfort of sunburned skin and calm itchiness. Pour 1 cup of apple cider vinegar into a warm tub of water and immerse yourself for 15 minutes.

The Milk and Honey Bath

Two cups of nonfat, instant milk and 1/2 cup of honey added to a warm bath will smooth and soften the skin.

The Buttermilk Bath

Mix together 1 cup of buttermilk, 3 tablespoons of Epsom salts, and 1/2 table-spoon of jojoba or canola oil and pour into the warm running water as the tub fills. This bath will soothe the skin.

Moisturizing Bath

Mix well 1 tablespoon of almond oil, 1 teaspoon liquid lecithin, 1 tablespoon of witch hazel extract, and 1 tablespoon of rose water. Massage into the skin and then step into a full tub of warm water.

The Herbal Bath

Put 1 cup of a dried herb or blend of dried herbs into a muslin bag or piece of cloth that has been secured with a piece of string or rubber band. Place this satchel of herbs in the tub as it fills with warm water.

For a relaxing bath: mix together 4 parts lavender, 2 parts rose, 4 parts chamomile, and 1 part hops.

For a stimulating bath: mix 2 parts peppermint, 1 part rosemary, 2 parts calendula, 1 part bay leaf and 1 part elderflower.

Salts Bath

Mix together 3/4 cup Epsom salts, 1/4 cup sea salt, and 1/4 cup baking soda. Pour into the tub as it is filling with water. This bath cleans, refreshes, and soft-ens the skin.

Stimulating

Stimulation increases the circulation of the blood and lymph to nourish and cleanse the skin. Stimulation can be done by dry brush massage, manual mas-sage, brisk drying with a rough terry towel, or using a washcloth with a grain meal scrub (not soap). Scrubs are exfoliating agents that can be used for the body (not the face) if they are gentle and the "texture" in them is from nut meals, grain meals, jojoba beads, coarse salt, or something similar with soft edges. (Do not use any product that uses sharp-edged substances such as walnut or almond shells.)

The best method to stimulate the skin is with a popular European technique called dry brush massage. Dry brush massage has been used for hundreds of years to benefit the skin as well as improve overall health. This technique cleans the skin without removing the protective pH mantle or natural skin oils. It stimulates the hormone and oil-producing glands in the dermal layer. By sloughing off the top layer of dead skin cells, dry brush massage opens the pores and assists the respirating function of the skin. It can assist in the breaking up of fat deposits and can smooth rough skin, especially on the upper arms, knees, and elbows. By stimulating circulation, it brings increased amounts of vital nutrients and oxygen to nourish the skin as well as underlying organs and tissues. Dry brush massage aids overall health by stimulating the lymphatic system and increasing the skin's ability as an eliminative organ.

Dry brush massage is best done before a bath or shower so the dead skin cells will be rinsed off the body. Use a long-handled, natural vegetable bristle brush that you use exclusively for this purpose. This type of brush is commonly available at natural food stores. Begin brushing the extremities (arms and legs) and work in circular motions toward the heart. Brush all of your skin, except the face. About once a month, wash the brush and let it dry thoroughly before using it again. Do not brush irritated skin, and be gentle with dry or sensitive skin. Dry brushing will leave you feeling warm and revitalized. Try it daily for remarkable results.

Conditioning/Nourishing

The skin is best nourished *internally* from the food we eat, the water we drink, and the air we breathe. However, *external* treatments can condition and nourish the skin as well. Because the skin is capable of absorbing substances with a sufficiently small molecular structure, there is value to well-formulated, nutritive body lotions, body oils, herbal wraps, and body packs. Just as these types of products are so carefully selected for the face, they also should be carefully selected for the body.

Custom-blended formulas to condition your skin can be easily made at home. Body oils of superb quality can be made by mixing 2 ounces of sweet almond, apricot kernel, or hazelnut oil with 25 drops of a single essential oil or a blend of essential oils. Essential oil of geranium and lavender are good for dehydrated skin (lacking water). Lavender, sandalwood, or rose are recommended for dry skin that is lacking oil. Bergamot and sandalwood are used for oily skin. Sensitive skin will be soothed by chamomile (Roman), neroli, or rose.

Body packs are also excellent for conditioning the skin. Similar in purpose to a facial mask, body packs can be made with a variety of ingredients and are best applied to clean skin after the pores have been relaxed from a warm bath or shower. A favorite pack is made with warmed honey, blended with a small amount of milk and then thickened with powdered oatmeal. A few drops of essential oils or herbal extract can also be added. Smooth the mixture on your skin and relax in an empty bathtub (or close all the blinds and do some housework) for about thirty minutes. Rinse off in the shower, first with warm water and then with cool. Pat dry. This body pack has a soothing, cleansing, and nutritive quality that is good for any skin type.

Another skin conditioning treatment is an herbal bath. Brew a strong tea, using one cup of dried herbs in three cups of water. For a wonderful bath blend for all types of skin, mix equal parts of comfrey leaves, chamomile, rose petals, and lavender. Pour the boiling water over the herbs and allow to steep, covered, for thirty minutes. Strain the herbs and then pour the tea into the bathtub full of warm water, stir well, and immerse yourself.

Protecting

Protection from environmental conditions is necessary to prevent skin irritation, damage, and moisture loss. The sun's damaging effects include burning, blistering, premature wrinkling, and skin cancer. Your skin can be protected from the sun by staying out of the sun, wearing a sunscreen or sunblock, and wearing protective clothing such as long sleeves, long pants, hats, and sunglasses. Excessive wind, salt water and air, extremes in temperature, and pollution can also cause dryness and damage, particularly for sensitive skin. The skin can be somewhat protected in these conditions with a good body lotion (or oil) and clothing, but it is best to try to *avoid over-exposure* to these situations.

Daily use of a body lotion or oil protects against moisture loss. It is best applied after a shower or bath because the skin has been hydrated and the oil will "seal in" the moisture. Apply a thin film, especially on the body parts exposed to the elements to help keep the skin soft and supple.

Exfoliating

Exfoliating the skin assists the sloughing off of dead skin cells on the surface. Our skin does this naturally. In fact, by the time we are seventy years old, we will have shed about forty pounds of dead skin cells. However, as we grow older there is more build-up of dead skin cells, and the sloughing-off process slows down. Exfoliating simply aids this natural process, revealing a softer, smoother skin. Dry brush massage is an excellent and effective method of exfoliation. (See above under "Stimulating.") Other mechanical methods are loofahs, scrubs, or pumice stones (for calloused areas only).

If you have sensitive skin and mechanical methods of exfoliation are too rough, green papaya is a gentle enzyme exfoliant that will help smooth and soften the skin by "digesting" dead skin cells. An alpha hydroxy acid product can also be used but is not as gentle as green papaya. (Both of these are described in more detail in Chapter 3, "Exfoliants.") These gentler types of exfoliants are excellent for sun-damaged or aging skin.

Special Care for the Hands

It has been said that the hands are not for ourselves—they are for others because they represent giving and receiving. The hands are one of our most important assets, so they deserve special care.

Because the hands are exposed to the elements and are almost constantly being used, they begin to show wear and tear and age sooner than other parts of the body. Following is a list of things you can do to help keep your hands soft and attractive and your nails in good condition.

1. Protect your hands from strong detergents and cleaning products by wearing rubber gloves. These chemicals can remove protective oils, and cause dryness and irritation as well as an allergic reaction.

2. Protect your hands and nails from frequent immersion in water. The skin can become dry and irritated. The nails, because they are capable of absorbing a small amount of water, swell when immersed. As they dry, they shrink back. This swelling and shrinking cycle makes the nails brittle.

3. Use a hand cream or lotion every time you wash your hands, and massage it well into the skin, the cuticles, and the nails. This will help prevent dryness, cracking, and brittleness.

4. To prevent "age spots" on the backs of your hands, keep them out of the sun and protect them with a sunblock of SPF 15.

5. Beware of nail cosmetics such as nail polishes. They are a frequent cause of allergic reactions, especially those that contain formaldehyde. The most common allergic reaction is a rash or itching around the nail, but some people have experienced the nail plate separating from the nail bed.

6. Do not use nail polish remover more than once a week. Using it too often will cause dryness to the nail and to surrounding tissue.

7. Protect the nail plate as well as the base of the nail from traumatic blows. Damage can result in permanently deformed nail growth.

8. After a bath or shower is an excellent time to groom your nails. Clean under the free edge, gently push back the cuticle while the skin is soft from bathing, and clip off any loose skin or hangnails.

9. Adequate amounts of protein, vitamins A and D, and the B vitamins are necessary for normal nail growth. Calcium, zinc, iodine, sulfur, and iron can also affect nail condition. Deficiencies may result in slow nail growth.

The nails are an appendage of the skin. They are a translucent plate that protects the tips of the fingers and toes and are composed mainly of a protein call keratin. The nail plate—the technical term for the nail itself—contains no nerves or blood vessels.

nail body or nail plate: the visible portion of the nail

nail bed: the portion of the skin upon which the nail body rests

free edge: the portion of the nail body which extends over the fingertips

nail matrix: the portion of the nail bed that extends beneath the skin. It contains nerves, lymph, and blood vessels. The matrix produces the nail, as its cells undergo a reproducing and hardening process.

lunula: the whitish half-moon that comes out from under the cuticle at the base of the nail plate

cuticle: the overlapping skin around the nail

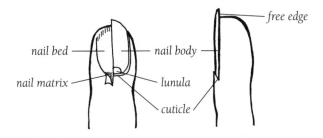

The At-Home Professional Manicure

Doing a manicure at home is fun, easy and inexpensive. Try to set the time aside once or twice a month to pamper your hands and nails.

Tools

1. A **nail file** (diamond files are the best but fine-grained emery boards will do).

2. An instrument or **nail brush** to clean under the free edge of the nail.

3. **Nippers** to trim off hangnails and loose skin around the nail.

4. **A nail buffer** (optional). This is a wonderful tool that will put a shine on the nail without polish.

5. **Orange wood stick** (available in most drug stores).

Supplies

1. **Essential oils** (singular or blends). Use lavender to soothe, relax, and relieve inflammation; chamomile (Roman) to soothe and soften the skin as well as relieve nervous tension; or peppermint to energize.

2. **Moisturizing lotion**

3. **Massage oil**

4. **Polish remover** (if necessary)

5. **Nail polish** (if desired, but not recommended)

6. **Castor oil**

The Manicure

1. Remove any nail polish.

2. Shape all your fingernails with the file. The professional way to file is from the outside corner of the nail towards the center—in one stroke and repeated until the nail is shaped to your preference. Sawing back and forth is not recommended because it shreds the nail and makes it prone to splitting.

3. Soak the fingertips in warm water. Add one or two drops of your favorite cosmetic essential oil such as lavender or geranium. Do not soak the nails in soapy water because it is drying to the nail and skin. The purpose of soaking is to soften the cuticle so that it can be gently pushed back— and plain water does this best. Soak for approximately ten minutes.

4. After soaking, take the edge of a towel and gently push the cuticle back. You can use the pad of your thumb (of the opposite hand) to do this. There are tools available for this purpose but they are not necessary unless you have not pushed your cuticles back for a long time. In that

case, you may need this special implement. Be certain it has soft rounded edges, and do not use excessive force.

5. In the process of pushing back the cuticle, small flaps of skin or hangnails may appear. If they do, snip them off with the nippers. Do not cut the cuticle itself. Cutting the cuticle may look good at first but it will cause hangnails in the following days.

6. Clean under the fingernail tip to remove dirt and nail filings.

7. Apply a small amount of castor oil to the cuticle and massage, while pushing it back.

8. Apply a moisturizing lotion and give yourself a thorough hand massage. Using the reflexology chart below, note the areas that you feel will benefit from extra attention. (For more information, see Chapter 18, "Reflexology.")

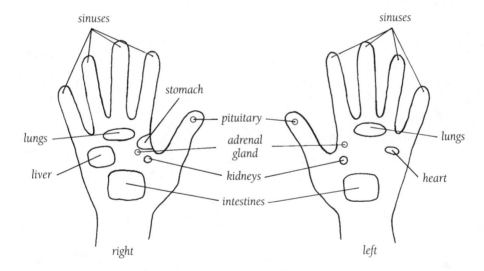

9. At this point, the manicure is finished, unless you choose to wear nail polish. If you do, you will need to clean the top of the nails with alcohol. This removes any oils left by the lotion so the polish will adhere well. Try to keep the alcohol on the nail plate only, avoiding the skin around the nails. Apply a base coat of polish, two coats of the color, and then finish with one or more coats of a top coat. As an alternative to polish, buff

the nail with a chamois nail buffer. This puts a natural sheen on the nail that won't chip!

Exercises for the Hands

These exercises are designed to stretch, tone and strengthen the hands as well as keep them flexible.

1. Put a rubber band around your fingertips then spread and relax your fingers against the band.

2. Try squeezing a tennis ball 15 times. This works the forearm muscles as well as the hand muscles. Increase the number of squeezes when the number you are doing becomes too easy. There are also devices sold at sports supply stores that are designed for this purpose.

3. Raise your arms overhead while inhaling, then count to 5 holding your breath and shake your hands vigorously from the wrists. Repeat 10 times.

4. Rotate each thumb and then tap each finger with the thumb for 10 rounds.

5. Tapping your nails on a table top and massaging the half-moon area can strengthen the nail by increasing circulation.

6. Stretch the fingers out, open and wiggle your fingers, and then clench your fist. Repeat for 5 rounds.

Interesting Facts About Hands and Nails

- Two of the largest areas of the brain are reserved for using the hands.

- During an average lifetime, fingers flex and extend about twenty-five million times.

- Compared to the use of legs or arms or feet, our hands almost never tire.

- The bones in both hands account for about one-fourth of all the bones in the body.

- The hands have thousands of nerve ending per square inch and they are especially concentrated in the fingertips.

- The palms have one of the richest supplies of sweat glands in the body and do not tan.

- Nails grow slower and become more brittle as we age.

- The technical terms for the fingers are: thumb-polex, pointer-index, middle-medius, ring-andularis, baby-ericularis.

- Women's nails are thinner than men's.

- Health changes or problems can be mirrored in the nails. Arthritis may cause thickening of the nail. Bluish nails may indicate a heart or lung problem. Pale nails may be a sign of anemia.

- Nails grow faster during warm weather and pregnancy. It is theorized that this is due to increased circulation during warm weather and hormonal changes during pregnancy.

- Nails are one of the toughest tissues of the body because they contain very little water—only about ten percent.

- Fingernails grow four times faster than toenails.

- It takes about 150 days to completely grow a new nail.

Recipes for Care of the Hands and Nails

Nail strengthening:
It is believed that a daily buffing and a periodic tapping of the nails on a hard surface will strengthen them.

To clean and whiten the nails:
Insert the fingertips into half a lemon and swish around, rinse, and pat dry.

Soapless hand cleanser:
Moisten the hands and massage with a handful of wheat or oat bran. Rinse and pat dry.

To hydrate the nails:
Soak the fingertips in warm water for five minutes and then massage with castor oil or a rich moisturizer.

Special Care For The Feet

Leonardo da Vinci said that the foot is the greatest engineering device in the world. Despite such accolades, feet are taken for granted by most people. As a result, most adult Americans suffer from foot problems at one time or another. Fortunately, many foot problems are preventable.

Preventing Foot Problems

1. Use your feet only for their intended purpose. Do not use them to kick doors, break wood, etc.

2. Wear socks to cushion the feet, cut down on friction, and to carry perspiration away from the foot. The socks should not have tight bands to constrict circulation.

3. Being overweight puts a tremendous strain on the skeletal and muscular structure of the foot. Try to stay at your optimum weight.

4. Buy the proper shoes to protect the feet from trauma and from heat and cold. Consider the fit, the material, and the function of the shoe before you buy. A proper fit means that there is a finger-width of space between the longest toe and the end of the shoe. The heel should fit snugly so it does not rub. There should be plenty of room in the toe area so your toes are not crammed together. This constricts circulation and can cause skin problems as well as damage to the muscles and joints. Your shoes should be made of either canvas or leather because these materials "breathe" and allow perspiration to evaporate. Always try on both shoes.

5. If you must stand on your feet all day, be certain your shoes fit properly and are low-heeled. They should have good arch support. Stand on a rubber mat, and if that is not possible, put sponge cushions in your shoes.

6. High-heeled shoes shorten your calf muscles, jam your toes, and shift your weight to the ball of the foot, which was not designed for this

purpose. If you must wear high heels, alternate them with lower-heeled shoes to help minimize the problems it may cause.

7. Try to go barefoot for a couple of hours every day so the feet can stretch and air out.

8. Learn to walk and stand with the feet parallel to each other—not turned in or out. This keeps the body's weight where it is meant to be—on the outside arch.

9. Clean the feet daily in a warm foot bath, then dry well between the toes and massage with a lotion to keep the skin soft.

10. Walk on grass, sand, or dirt as often as you can to exercise the feet and retain good foot structure.

11. Try to avoid wearing the same pair of shoes two days in a row. It is important to let the shoes dry and air out to extend the life of the shoe and to help prevent bacterial growth.

At-Home Professional Pedicure

Tools & Supplies

The same tools and supplies are required for the pedicure as for the manicure (see "Special Care for the Hands" in this chapter). In addition, sturdy nail clippers (designed for toenails) and a pumice stone will be needed.

The Pedicure

1. Remove any nail polish.

2. Soak your feet for about ten minutes in a warm foot bath. Soaking cleanses the feet and softens rough, dry skin. It also relieves muscle tension.

3. Pat your feet dry and clip the toenails. Toenails are much coarser than fingernails and will cut easier after they have soaked in water. If you have any sharp or rough edges left on the nail after clipping, you can file them. Remember, NEVER clip into the corners of the toenails—it can cause an ingrown nail.

4. Gently pumice any dry, rough, or calloused areas. Do this to remove only the tough outer skin. Do not try to completely remove a callus. It has developed there to protect an area that needs it. If you remove the whole callus, you may find the area very sore and the callus will rebuild again.

5. Clean under the free edge of the nail on all toes.

6. Using an orange wood stick, very gently push back all the cuticles a little bit.

7. Clip any loose skin or hangnails but do not clip the cuticle itself.

8. Massage each cuticle with a small amount of castor oil, pushing the cuticle back as you massage.

9. Using a moisturizing lotion or aromatherapy massage oil, give yourself a generous foot massage. Refer to the reflexology chart below for added benefits.

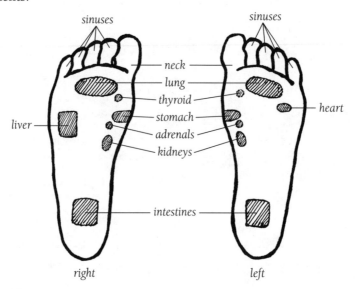

10. Remove any excess oil or lotion with a towel or tissue.

11. If polishing is desired, follow the same procedure as for the fingernails.

Exercises for the Feet

1. Stand on your toes, tip-toed, hold for ten seconds, then put your heels on the ground. Repeat. This stretches the muscles and the heel cord and strengthens the calf muscles. It also helps to develop good balance.

2. Walking on the outer edge of your feet while barefoot will stretch muscles and strengthen the ankles.

3. While seated, pick up marbles with your toes (barefooted) and drop them into a cup. This develops coordination, strengthens muscles, flexes the ankle, and stimulates the leg muscles.

4. While seated, with bare feet, curl your toes under your feet. Feel the stretching in the top of the foot and in the toes. Hold for a while and then repeat.

5. This exercise is one of the best: Walk barefoot on a sandy beach. This will strengthen all the muscles in the foot and the calf.

6. While sitting, extend your feet in front of you. Point and flex your feet ten times.

Recipes for Care of the Feet

Cooling Foot Massage Oil:
Mix 4 drops of essential oil of peppermint into two ounces of olive oil. Massage the feet.

Foot Soak #1:
Add one tablespoon of baking soda to the container of soaking water. This will help to loosen dead skin, which can then be pumiced off.

Foot Soak #2:
Add 1/4 cup apple cider vinegar to your foot bath. This will relieve itching and invigorate the skin.

Exfoliating Foot Massage Blend:

Blend equal parts of Epsom salt, table salt, and bicarbonate of soda. Soak feet for ten minutes in warm water and massage well with the blend. Rinse well and then soak again for a few minutes.

Relieve Foot Fatigue:

Add a couple of drops of essential oil of rosemary to your foot bath. A few drops of lavender essential oil are also effective.

Foot Skin Softener:

Mash an avocado and mix it with the juice of half a lemon, one tablespoon of castor oil, and one tablespoon of jojoba oil. Massage this into the feet and then cover with a pair of socks overnight. In the morning, rinse your feet well and scrub the rough areas with a nail brush.

An Herb Bath for Tired Feet:

Mix 1 part thyme, 2 parts rosemary, 3 parts peppermint, and 2 parts chamomile (Roman). Infuse 4 tablespoons of the herb blend in 2 cups of boiling water and steep for 15 minutes. Strain and then add to the foot bath.

Foot Bath to Relieve Odor:

Mix 1/4 cup of apple cider vinegar with 8 drops of essential oil of sage, cypress, or bergamot (or a combination of these) into a warm foot bath. Add 1/4 cup baking soda and stir to dissolve. Soak your feet for 15 minutes.

6

Natural Ingredients for Skin Care

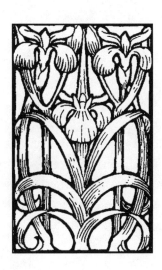

*N*ature has given us a magnificent and broad spectrum of valuable resources for ingredients in natural cosmetics. Herbal extracts from plants, essential oils distilled from flowers, rich and emollient plant oils, and botanicals from the sea are examples of nature's gifts that can be used in formulations to nurture and rejuvenate the complexion.

When you shop for skin care products, read the labels and look for the following natural ingredients. They can be found in all types of skin care products such as cleansers, toners, moisturizers, masks, and facial misters. When shopping, it is helpful to bring a cosmetic ingredient book such as Ruth Winter's *A Consumer's Dictionary of Cosmetic Ingredients,* or Natalia Michalun's *Skin Care and Cosmetic Ingredients Dictionary* so you can look up information on unfamiliar ingredients. Some have names that appear very foreign and "chemicalized." Do not judge these too quickly as ingredients to be avoided. After you look them up in the ingredients book, you may discover that they are fine to use.

Aloe Vera is a tropical plant whose sharp-edged, triangular leaves contain a viscous, transparent gel that when used externally promotes healing and cellular renewal. Aloe vera is well known for its therapeutic value for burns. The gel contains amino acids, minerals, vitamins, carbohydrates, and enzymes. Components of the gel are believed to easily penetrate the skin, carrying nutrients into the deeper layers. Aloe vera is soothing, moisturizing, and toning for all types of skin. It has the ability to balance the complexion—helping to bring moisture to dry skin and controlling oily skin. It is excellent for blemished skin due to its antibiotic, anti-bacterial, and anti-inflammatory qualities.

Alpha Hydroxy Acids (AHAs) are a group of compounds found in a variety of food sources. Glycolic acid is the most widely used in skin care products and is most commonly derived from sugar cane. However, the other alpha hydroxy acids in the group—such as lactic (from sour milk), tartaric (from grapes), citric (from citrus fruits), and malic (from apples)—are finding their way into use as well. Alpha hydroxy acids improve the feel and appearance of the skin by loosening and dissolving a glue-like protein that binds the dead skin cells (corneocytes) on

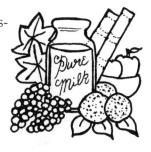

the surface of the skin. As these dead skin cells are loosened and fall away, a smoother and younger-appearing complexion is revealed. The regular use of alpha hydroxy acids has been shown to soften fine lines and wrinkles, improve dry skin, help control blemishes, and reduce the discoloration commonly referred to as "age spots."

Clay, known as nature's detoxifier, has the ability to absorb toxins, to cleanse, and to deodorize. Clay is rich in mineral content and is most frequently used in facial masks to increase circulation, nourish, detoxify, and revitalize the skin. It also has natural antiseptic properties. Clay is non-toxic and not a known allergen.

Essential Oils are concentrated extracts from specific plants. As a group, they are one of the most active natural ingredients in skin care today. Favorite cosmetic essential oils include carrot seed, cedarwood, chamomile (Roman), clary sage, frankincense, geranium, jasmine, lavender, lemon, neroli, patchouli, rose, rosemary, rosewood, sandalwood, tea tree, and ylang ylang. These essential oils are discussed in greater detail in Chapter 9, "Aromatherapy."

Glycerin is a natural humectant (the ability to attract and hold moisture). Derived from animal or vegetable fats, glycerin is used in cosmetics to hold moisture next to the skin to relieve dryness. It also aids in the spreadability of a product. Glycerin, when formulated in high percentages, may be undesirable because it can attract moisture *from* the skin, which could lead to dryness, so cosmetic products should contain less than twenty percent. In addition, too much glycerin in a product will make it feel sticky.

Green Papaya is rich in a proteolytic (protein-digesting) enzyme called papain that, when used on the skin, dissolves and digests old, dead skin cells without harming younger, living cells. This gentle exfoliation process reveals a softer smoother skin. Papain is most potent while

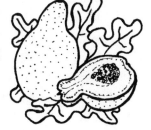

the papaya fruit is still green. Green papaya has also been shown to be effective in neutralizing free radicals, perhaps due to its high vitamin A & C content.

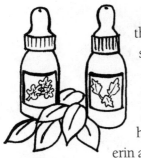 **Herbal Extracts** have been used in skin care cosmetics for thousands of years for their ability to soften, soothe, protect, stimulate, and rejuvenate the skin. Vitamins, trace minerals, amino acids, and enzymes can be found in herbs, providing effective, active ingredients for beautifying the complexion. Herbal extracts are made by extracting the properties of the herb with a solvent, usually water or alcohol, although glycerin and vinegar are also used. Many herbs are used in cosmetics. Listed below are some of the most popular.

Arnica soothes skin irritation as it purifies and promotes healing.

Calendula cleanses, soothes, and promotes healing. It also reduces inflammation and stimulates circulation.

Chamomile reduces inflammation, soothes, and accelerates healing. It softens the skin and promotes the regeneration of skin cells.

Comfrey is used to soothe and heal because of its allantoin and carotene content. It also cleanses, moisturizes, reduces inflammation, and promotes the regeneration of cells. Comfrey has an astringent quality.

Elderflower cleanses, reduces inflammation and acts as a mild astringent.

Ginkgo biloba reduces inflammation and increases circulation and cellular activity. It is a powerful anti-oxidant.

Ginseng tones, rejuvenates, balances, and has anti-oxidant qualities. It may also stimulate the formation of new cells.

Green tea extract is used as an anti-inflammatory, anti-irritant and anti-oxidant.

Horsetail is rich in silica, a mineral necessary for healthy skin and hair. It also has astringent properties and is toning to the skin.

Lavender balances and promotes cellular regeneration and rapid healing.

Nettle purifies and tones. It is rich in minerals and stimulates circulation.

Peppermint purifies and has astringent qualities.

Rose soothes and harmonizes the skin and is good for all skin types.

Rosemary stimulates circulation, rejuvenates, and tones. It also has antiseptic and anti-oxidant properties.

St. Johnswort is used to tone, strengthen, and heal. It has a calming quality.

Witch Hazel acts as an astringent and reduces inflammation.

Yarrow has slight astringent qualities and is toning to the skin.

Honey has been used for thousands of years for food, medicine, and cosmetics. It is 98% sugar and 2% enzymes, vitamins, and minerals. Honey has a stimulating and toning effect on the skin and is a mild antiseptic. It is a natural humectant and bacteria will not grow in it. Both of these factors make honey a valuable component for moisturizing formulations. The darker honeys are better for skin care because they contain more minerals.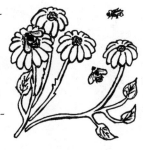

Hyaluronic Acid is a mucopoly-saccharide (complex carbohydrate) that is a gel-like natural component of human skin. In the dermal layer, collagen and elastin are surrounded by hyaluronic acid, and its water-binding quality helps maintain moisture and flexibility in the skin. The percentage of hyaluronic acid in the skin is directly related to the moisture content in the intercellular environment of the dermis. Hyaluronic acid can hold a thousand times its own weight in water and has the ability to hold that moisture for days. Even after a week, it still retains ten times its weight in water. These capabilities are unprecedented and make hyaluronic acid an exceptional humectant and moisturizer in skin care products, relieving dryness and helping to prevent the formation of fine lines and wrinkles. The hyaluronic acid that is used in cosmetics was originally derived from rooster's combs; now, it is being bio-engineered and plant sources have been developed.

Natural Colors are used by some natural cosmetic manufacturers to replace artificial Food, Drug & Cosmetics (FD&C) colors in all types of skin care products and make-up. Artificial FD&C colors, suspected carcinogens, are known to cause allergic reaction in sensitive people, and they may have an impact on the environment by adversely affecting animals and the food chain. In addition, artificial colors have been tested on animals for certification. Many consumers concerned about animals, the environment, and their health are choosing to use products that contain only natural color pigments. The most common natural color pigments are beet powder, beta carotene, minerals (iron oxides), grape skin extract, chlorophyll, turmeric, carmine, and annatto. Natural coloring pigments do not require animal testing and are not suspected to cause health problems or allergic reactions.

Oat, a natural cereal grain, is rich in vitamins and minerals and has the best balance of amino acids of all cereal proteins. Used in cosmetics, oats soothe sensitive skin, moisturize dry skin, and relieve itching, irritation and inflammation. Oat bran is used as a thickener and moisturizer. Beta glucan, which is extracted from the oat bran is used as a humectant, capable of penetrating the skin for deep moisturizing. Oat flour is a natural emulsifier for skin care products and can also be used for pressed powders. Oat starch is used in baby powders and deodorants to replace talc. Oat protein, rich in amino acids, moisturizes and is used in both skin and hair care products.

Plant Oils, historically, were the first cosmetic ingredients to be in constant demand, and were used extensively to make soap, cold creams, and lotions. There was a period of time when their use in cosmetic formulations diminished because of their expense and limited shelf life. Today, however, natural oils are back in use and are valued for their emollient, nourishing, soothing, and moisturizing benefits to the skin. The following plant oils have exceptional value for cosmetic use.

Almond oil (sweet) is extracted from almond nutmeats and contains vitamins, minerals, fatty acids, and protein. This lightweight oil is a soothing emollient and skin softener. It is also nourishing and revitalizing and used to relieve dryness, itching, and inflammation. Almond oil is excellent for all types of skin but especially mature, dry, or sensitive. Almond oil has a short shelf life, so purchase only what you can use in a few months and keep it refrigerated.

Apricot kernel oil is a smooth, lightweight oil high in vitamin A and rich in minerals. It has a very nice texture and is good for all skin types, especially sensitive and mature.

Avocado oil is a nutritive oil that contains vitamins A, D, and E, protein, lecithin, and fatty acids. It is a superb emollient with some sunscreen properties. Avocado oil is easily absorbed into the skin. It smooths and softens and is good for all skin types, especially dry or mature.

Borage seed oil is rich in essential fatty acids and contains vitamins and minerals. It is a regenerative oil and is good for all skin types, especially mature.

Canola oil contains essential fatty acids, vitamins and minerals. It is good for all skin types and is easily absorbed into the skin.

Castor oil is a remarkable healing oil that is believed to boost the immune system and help prevent scarring. It is non-drying and best diluted and used only in small amounts in a base oil for cosmetic purposes. Castor oil is good for dry and chapped skin.

Coconut oil is excellent to relieve dry, itchy skin. It is a semi-solid at room temperature and quickly melts when applied to the skin.

Flax seed oil is one of the richest sources of essential fatty acids. It is wonderful for all skin types and is especially beneficial taken internally as a supplement. It is rich in natural vitamin E, which provides anti-oxidant qualities.

Hazelnut oil is a gentle, lightweight oil that is very compatible with the skin and leaves no greasy residue. It contains vitamins, minerals, fatty acids, and protein. Hazelnut oil is good for all skin types, especially dry or damaged skin. It stimulates circulation and has a slight astringent action. Hazelnut oil is frequently used as a base for essential oil blends.

Jojoba oil, derived from the bean of a desert bush, is excellent for the skin to soothe, moisturize, and nurture. Jojoba is said to closely resemble the natural oil of our skin and has the unique quality of being a liquid wax, which helps prevent rancidity. Jojoba oil contains minerals and protein. It is non-greasy and is easily absorbed into the skin as it nourishes, lubricates, and softens.

Lanolin is an excellent emollient oil from sheep's wool and a superb moisturizer. The sheep are not harmed to obtain the lanolin.

Kukui nut oil is from the kukui nut of Hawaii. This light and easily absorbed oil is high in essential fatty acids and has the ability to smooth, soothe, and soften the skin. It is especially good for irritated, dry, or chapped skin.

Macadamia nut oil is rich in monounsaturated oils, oleic and palmitoleic acid. It is excellent for all types of skin, especially dry and mature because of the palmitoleic acid—a substance found in the sebum of young skin. As the skin ages, the amount of palmitoleic acid decreases.

Neem oil is from the neem tree, a tall evergreen common in India where it is considered sacred. It is healing and strengthening to the skin with antiseptic, and anti-inflammatory qualities.

Olive oil is rich in vitamins and minerals and contains some protein. Nourishing and calming to the skin, olive oil is believed to have both disinfecting and wound-healing capabilities.

Peanut oil is a heavy, polyunsaturated oil and is excellent for dry skin.

Rosehip seed oil is high in essential fatty acids. It is believed to be a tissue regenerator and has been used to help heal burns and sunburns, to improve acne scars, and to reduce wrinkles.

Safflower oil is a nutritive oil that is easily absorbed into the skin. It is recommended for oilier skin types.

Sesame oil, pressed from the sesame seed, is rich in vitamins and minerals and contains some proteins and lecithin. It is believed to provide some protection from the rays of the sun. Sesame oil is good for all skin types.

Shea butter (also known as karite) is extracted from the fruit of a tree found in Africa. It contains allantoin, known for its healing abilities, and is traditionally used for a variety of skin problems such as eczema, sunburn, and dermatitis. It is also used for aching muscles. Shea butter can protect the skin from environmental damage and is gentle and safe to use even on sensitive, fragile skin.

Soybean oil is a good base for massage oil. It is nutritive and contains vitamins and lecithin.

Squalene used in cosmetics was originally derived from the liver of a shark. Now, it is available from olives which provide a more abundant, less expensive, and odorless source. Squalene is extremely compatible with the skin—it has a molecular structure that is similar to the squalene that is secreted by the skin's oil glands (approximately ten percent of sebum is squalene). Squalene is good for all skin types, especially dry and sensitive, to protect and lubricate. It easily penetrates the skin as it helps to accelerate new cell growth and leaves the skin feeling soft and smooth. Squalene also helps the skin retain moisture and can bring relief to dry and delicate skin. It does not clog pores, does not leave an oily residue on the skin, and is not known to cause allergic reactions or skin sensitivities.

Sunflower oil is rich in linoleic acid (an essential fatty acid) and light in texture. It contains vitamins and minerals and some lecithin.

Wheat germ oil is a heavy oil rich in lecithin, vitamin E, vitamin A, essential fatty acids, and protein. It is highly nutritive and easily penetrates the skin to moisturize, regenerate, and nourish. Wheat germ oil is soothing and healing and good for all skin types, especially dry and aging skin. Due to wheat germ oil's strong odor, it is generally used in formulations in low percentages.

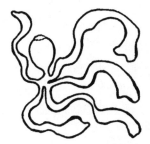

Sea Plants contain an abundance of vitamins, minerals, and amino acids. Seaweed is believed to contain nature's most complete and balanced source of nutrients—there are more than ninety different elements found in seaweed that are essential to the human body. Sea vegetation conditions and hydrates the skin while it remineralizes, nourishes, and rejuvenates. It also has free-radical scavenging and detoxifying capabilities. One theory about why sea plants are so good for the skin is that their chemical composition is similar to that of plasma in the human body. This enables particularly good penetration of the nutrients. The mineral salts are easily absorbed by skin cells, allowing the cells to hold on to their own moisture, making the skin soft and more supple. Alginates found in seaweeds make the skin more flexible and elastic. Sea plants oxygenate and invigorate the skin tissues, and when combined with other ingredients, assist in their penetration.

Titanium Dioxide is a white mineral used as a coloring agent, a sunscreen, and a sunblock. Titanium dioxide physically reflects UVA, UVB, and UVC rays from the sun and helps prevent skin cancers and premature wrinkling of the skin. It is safe, non-toxic, non-irritating, and not known to cause allergic reactions.

Vinegar is made from a variety of sources such as apples, rice, wine, or malt. Natural apple cider vinegar is the best for skin care and is especially good to restore the pH balance of the skin. It also soothes and softens.

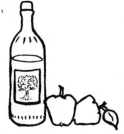

Vitamins are defined as "a group of chemically unrelated organic (carbon containing) nutrients that are essential in small quantities for normal metabolism, growth, and physical well-being."[1] The vitamins used in cosmetics are used primarily for their anti-oxidant, free-radical scavenging capabilities and their rejuvenating properties. Listed here are the most popular.

Vitamin A is necessary for tissue generation, repair, and maintenance. It accelerates the formation of new cells, prevents increased keratinization (thickening) of the skin, deters excessive dryness, and regulates glandular functions in the skin. It also has anti-oxidant properties.

Vitamin C is an excellent anti-oxidant that protects skin cells. It fights infections and supports collagen production.

Vitamin D is used for smoothing the skin and its anti-aging properties.

Vitamin E's most valuable contribution in skin care is its ability to slow down the aging and degeneration of skin cells. It promotes cellular renewal, skin elasticity, and healing. Its superb anti-oxidant qualities fight free radicals both in the skin and on the skin surface and help to keep cosmetic products fresh.

Vitamin F (essential fatty acids) is excellent for the hydration and lubrication of skin cells. It helps to keep the skin soft, smooth, and youthful.

Panthenol (pro-vitamin B-5) is used to moisturize the skin. It is soothing, nourishing, and aids in tissue repair and cellular regeneration.

Pycnogenol, though not a true vitamin, is a flavonoid from the bark of the French maritime pine tree and is a powerful anti-oxidant. Pycnogenol is also found in beans, grapes, cranberries, and other fruits and vegetables. Its anti-oxidant qualities are believed to be more active than both vitamin E and vitamin C. In the dermal layer of the skin pycnogenol strengthens capillary walls and binds to collagen to help prevent wrinkles and environmental damage to the skin.

Water is one of the most important ingredients in a cosmetic formula for the skin because moisture is the key to keeping skin youthful and healthy, soft and supple. Water is used in creams and lotions as part of the emulsion (water and oil combined). Water also helps carry active ingredients into the skin.

7

Making Your Own
Skin Care Products

Cleansers
Aromatherapy Facial Oils
Facial Misters

Toners
Masks
Massage Oils

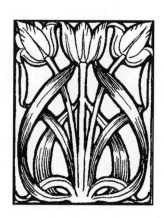

igh-quality, natural skin care products were not always as available as they are today. So in the past, those people who wanted only purity and excellence to touch their skins made their own products. Though simply purchasing skin care products at your local health food store is more convenient, it is not as much fun and not nearly as rewarding as making your own. If you have never tried creating a special toner or bath oil, perhaps this chapter will encourage you to experiment with nature's bounty.

Home-made cosmetics have distinct advantages over store-bought products. The cosmetics are fresh with no compromising ingredients such as preservatives, artificial colors, or artificial fragrances. The products can be designed to meet your specific needs and preferences. You also have control over the quality of the ingredients, how the product is made, and how it is stored. In other words, you have complete control over the end product. An added bonus: Home-made cosmetics are less expensive because there is no added cost of packaging, advertising, and distributing.

Categories of Ingredients for Skin Care Products

There are four categories of ingredients, detailed below, that are most frequently and successfully used to make skin care products at home. They are foods, herbs, plant oils, and vitamins. Remember to keep your home-made cosmetics refrigerated because they do not have preservatives. Replace them with a fresh batch when needed.

Foods

Fresh food such as strawberries, avocadoes, carrots, and eggs are nutritious and healthful foods to eat. They are also valuable ingredients in skin care products. Common foods that can be used for cosmetic preparations are:

Almonds can be ground into meal or flour and used for cleansing grains. They refine the pores, and help combat roughness and dryness.

Apple is used in facial masks and lotions to combat dryness and blemishes. It softens the skin and acts as an astringent. The juice is soothing if it is made from the entire apple and is good for all skin types, especially sensitive and fair skin.

Apricot refines and smooths the skin. It has a high carotene content (vitamin A) and is good for all skin types.

Avocado is used in facials to cleanse, nourish, and relieve dryness. It has excellent penetrating qualities and contains vitamins A, D, and E and the minerals potassium and sulfur.

Banana is used in facial masks for normal to dry skin. It is high in potassium and contains some vitamin C. Bananas are very nourishing and can soothe, soften, and smooth the texture of the skin.

Barley (cooked) is excellent in facial masks to help prevent wrinkles and pimples. Ground barley can be used as a granular cleanser, and barley water may be used as a facial wash to relieve dry, itchy skin.

Bran (wheat) is used as a cleanser for the face and hands. It is nourishing and softening and can be used in masks to combat large pores and dryness. It contains iron, potassium, and B vitamins.

Carrot (steamed and ground) is excellent used in facial masks to help clear pimples and unclog pores. It is a general skin tonic because of the high vitamin A content and good for all skin types, especially dry.

Cantaloupe is superb for skin that is lacking moisture.

Cornmeal can be used as an exfoliating scrub for non-sensitive skin areas such as the elbows and feet.

Cucumber has a cleansing, cooling and toning effect on the skin. Cold cucumber slices over the eyes can help to reduce puffiness. The juice of the whole cucumber has an enzyme that softens the skin. Cucumber is good for normal and dry skins.

Egg is used in facial masks. The yolk is rich in oils that are good to combat skin dryness. The whites of the egg are used in masks for pore tightening, to reduce puffiness, and to soothe sunburn.

Grape is used to moisturize and nourish the skin and is especially good for sensitive skin.

Lemon is very acidic, so it is useful whenever a lower pH is required. Lemon has astringent, antiseptic, and bleaching qualities and is used in facial masks and lotions for blackheads, oiliness, and large pores. Lemon also removes stains from the nails and hands.

Milk (whole) is excellent used alone as a facial cleanser. Milk cleans, softens, and nourishes. It is good for all skin types and useful in foot baths. Milk can also be used to infuse herbs.

Oats and oatmeal have cleansing, softening, nutritive and soothing qualities. Oat flour is used in cleansers, and cooked oatmeal is excellent in facial masks.

Onion is used in facial masks for blemished skin.

Orange is used to soften and cleanse the skin. It is best suited for normal and oily skins.

Papaya contains enzymes that act as a gentle exfoliant on the skin. It is high in vitamin A and C. Papaya can be used under the eyes to reduce dark circles and as a gentle facial cleanser. It is good for all skin types.

Parsley (juice) is used as a healing lotion for skin blemishes.

Peach is used to refine and smooth the skin. Good for all skin types, peach contains some vitamin A and C.

Pear is used to moisturize and refresh; it is good for normal skin.

Pineapple is used in facial masks for its rejuvenating qualities and enzyme activity. It can clear the complexion and is best suited for normal skin.

Potato is used to reduce puffiness and soothe burns for all skin types.

Strawberry is used in facial masks for its ability to gently soften, moisturize, and nourish. Strawberries are used primarily for normal and oily skins. Some skin may have an allergic reaction to strawberries. To lessen this risk, crush strawberries in milk or yogurt prior to applying to the skin.

Sweet cream can be used in facials to minimize wrinkles and dry skin. It is very soothing.

Tomatoes have a cleansing, nourishing, and stimulating effect on the skin. They are acidic and rich in vitamins A and C. Tomatoes can be used in masks or lotions and are excellent for oily skin. They are not recommended for sensitive or very dry skin.

Yogurt is used in facial masks on oily or dull skin to nourish and cleanse.

Herbs

Herbs in cosmetic preparations play an important and versatile role. They soothe, stimulate, moisturize, tighten, heal, and cleanse the skin. Herbs may be used alone, blended with other herbs, or combined with other ingredients in the form of tinctures, teas, or oils. See Chapter 6, "Herbal Extracts" for a list of the most popular cosmetics herbs.

Plant Oils

When used in cosmetic preparations, plant oils have the ability to cleanse, moisturize, and soothe the skin while providing nourishment and protection. Oils can be used alone, in combination with other oils, infused with herbs, or combined with food ingredients. Plant oils are rich in essential and non-essential fatty acids, which are necessary for general good health, and especially for smooth, soft, supple skin. Oils are best kept refrigerated because of their tendency to become rancid. (Rancidity is a chemical change in a fat or oil that is a process of deterioration resulting from the combination of oxygen from the air with the unsaturated fatty acids in the oil.) For a list of valuable cosmetic oils and their attributes, see Chapter 6, "Plant Oils."

Vitamins

Vitamins in skin care products are used primarily for their anti-oxidant and re-juvenating capabilities. See Chapter 6, "Vitamins" for a list of important cosmetic vitamins and their uses.

The Recipes

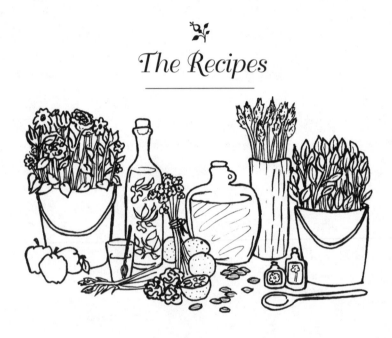

Cleansers

to cleanse the skin of soil without removing protective oils

Herbal Milk Cleanser (*for all skin types*)

To make: Soak 1 heaping tablespoon of a dried herb or herb blend in a cup of cold, whole, raw milk for a couple of hours. Strain and refrigerate the milk.

To use: Rinse your face with warm water. Shake the milk cleanser, and dip a cotton ball in the milk, and wipe your face. You may need to use more than one cotton ball. Rinse with warm water and follow with a cool-water splash.

This is a true milk cleanser. Milk cleansers as we know them in commercial products are an emulsion of water and oil. Whole milk, with the fat globules throughout, also provides this water-and-oil mix. (This cleanser will not remove water-resistant make-up).

To custom-make an herbal cleansing milk for specific skin types, use the following herbal combinations:

Normal: equal parts comfrey leaf, lavender, rose, rosemary

Oily: equal parts yarrow, lavender, lemon peel, witch hazel, comfrey leaf

Dry: equal parts chamomile, comfrey leaf, rosemary, elderflower

Sensitive: equal parts rose, chamomile

Blemished: equal parts lavender, licorice, comfrey, chamomile, sage

Mature: equal parts chamomile, lavender, comfrey leaf, orange blossom, rose

Granular Cleanser #1 *(for normal, combination, and dry skin)*

To make: Mix equal parts finely ground oatmeal (oat flour), wheat bran, and honey. Mix in small amounts of olive oil and apple cider vinegar to make a paste and a couple of drops of lavender essential oil or essential oil of your choice.

To use: Rinse your face with warm water. Apply cleanser and gently hug and press the skin with slight massage. Rinse well with warm water followed by a cool-water splash.

Granular Cleanser #2 *(for normal, combination, and dry skin)*

To make: Mix 1 part finely ground almonds or almond flour, 1 part oat flour, and 1 part finely ground herb blend (rose, lavender, and comfrey leaf in equal parts).

To use: Put 1 tablespoon of this dry mixture in the palm of your hand and mix with sweet almond oil, water, milk, or aloe vera to form a paste. Work gently over moistened skin. Do not scrub.

Gentle Scrub Cleanser #1 *(for all skin types except sensitive)*

To make: Mix whole milk with enough wheat germ to form a paste. Add a small amount of honey and mix well.

To use: Rinse your face with warm water. Apply cleanser and gently massage over the skin with patting and pressing motions. Rinse well with warm water followed by a cool-water splash.

Gentle Scrub Cleanser #2 (*for all skin types except sensitive*)

To make: Mix herbal milk or plain cream with enough oat flour to form a paste. Let sit for a few minutes as the oatmeal softens.

To use: Rinse your face with warm water. Apply cleanser and gently massage over the skin with patting and pressing motions. Rinse well with warm water followed by a cool-water splash.

Granular Almond Cleanser (*for normal, dry, combination, or mature skin*)

To make: Make a paste of fine almond flour, honey, a little apple cider vinegar, and olive oil.

To use: Work gently over a moist face and rinse well.

Clay Cleanser (*for normal, oily, or combination skin*)

To make: Mix 4 tablespoons of clay, and 1 tablespoon each of powdered lavender and comfrey leaf.

To use: Mix approximately 1 teaspoon of the clay-and-herbs mixture with enough water to make a paste. Gently apply to the face and neck with light massage. Rinse with warm water followed by a cool water splash.

Optional: Add 2 drops of essential oil of geranium, ylang ylang, or rosewood when you mix the dry blend with water.

Easy Make-up Remover and Cleanser
(*for normal, dry, combination, sensitive, or mature skin*)

To use: Apply any vegetable or fruit oil such as olive oil or apricot kernel oil to the skin and gently pat, press, and lightly massage. Rinse with warm water followed by a cool-water splash.

Make-up Remover

To make: Mix 2 tablespoons milk and 1 teaspoon vegetable oil

To use: Put in a container and shake vigorously. Apply with wash cloth or cotton ball.

Miscellaneous Ingredients for Cleansers

grain flours (such as oat or barley)	clay	essential oils	powdered herbs
nut flours (such as almond)	oils	spirulina	herbal extracts
seed flours (such as or sunflower)	honey	salt	

Toners

to remove all traces of cleanser and to condition the skin

Lavender Toner (*for all skin types*)

To make: Add 4 drops of essential oil of lavender to 1/2 cup of water.

To use: Shake well before use. After the skin has been cleansed, dampen a cotton ball and apply to the face with a wiping motion.

Lemon Toner and Astringent (*for normal, oily, or combination skin*)

To make: Squeeze and strain the juice of one lemon. Mix with 1/2 to 1 cup of water, depending on the desired strength.

To use: Apply to clean face using a cotton ball and a wiping motion.

Aloe Vera Juice Toner (*for normal, oily, combination, or blemished skin*)

To use: Dampen cotton ball and apply to clean skin with a wiping motion. Aloe vera is especially good for blemished skin. Leave on for a few minutes and then rinse your face with cool water and gently pat dry. The very clear, almost liquid aloe vera juice can be left on. Dry, sensitive, and aging skins may be able to use aloe vera juice as a toner, but in some cases the aloe is too drying. In this case, it can be diluted 50/50 with water.

Vinegar Toner (*for all skin types*)

To make: Apple cider vinegar diluted with water makes an excellent skin toner and conditioner. Use 2 tablespoons of vinegar to 1 cup of water. This proportion can be adjusted for various skin types such as increasing the amount of water for sensitive skin or decreasing the amount for oily skin.

To use: Dampen a cotton ball and apply to clean skin with a wiping motion.

Herbal Tea Toners (*for all skin types*)

To make: Pour 1 cup of boiling water over 1 to 3 teaspoons of your favorite herb or blend of herbs and steep for one hour. Strain. Mix with 1 tablespoon of apple cider vinegar (optional). Store in refrigerator and make fresh every week.

To use: Dampen a cotton ball and apply to clean skin with a wiping motion. For suggested herbal combinations, see "Herbal Milk Cleanser" in the beginning of this chapter.

Aromatherapy Facial Oils

essential oils in a nutritive base to nourish and rejuvenate

Base Oil Blends for Aromatherapy Facial Oils

#1 Mix 1 part apricot kernel oil, 1 part almond oil, and 1/4 part olive oil.

#2 Mix 3 parts sweet almond oil, 1 part olive oil, and 1/8 jojoba oil.

#3 Mix 2 parts jojoba oil, 2 parts hazelnut oil, and 1 part sweet almond oil.

#4 Mix 1 part jojoba oil and 2 parts sweet almond oil.

#5 Especially for mature skin: Mix 3 parts kukui nut oil, 1 part macadamia nut oil, 1 part jojoba oil, 1/2 part avocado oil, and 1/8 part calendula oil.

Use 2 ounces of a base oil blend with 25 drops of essential oils. (If the skin is very sensitive, use less essential oils.)

Aromatherapy Facial Oil for Normal Skin #1

1/4 ounce jojoba oil

3/4 ounce sweet almond oil

8 drops lavender

4 drops chamomile (Roman)

Aromatherapy Facial Oil for Normal Skin #2

1/2 ounce jojoba oil

1/2 ounce hazelnut oil

1 teaspoon sweet almond oil

6 drops lavender

2 drops rosewood

4 drops geranium

Aromatherapy Facial Treatment for Oily Skin #1

1 ounce aloe vera juice

1 teaspoon witch hazel

8 drops lavender

2 drops ylang ylang

2 drops cypress

Shake vigorously before applying.

Aromatherapy Facial Treatment for Oily Skin #2

1 ounce aloe vera juice

1 teaspoon witch hazel

3 drops geranium

6 drops lavender

2 drops clary sage

1 drop juniper

Shake vigorously before applying.

Aromatherapy Facial Oil for Dry Skin #1

1/2 ounce jojoba oil

1/2 ounce sweet almond oil

1/2 teaspoon flaxseed oil

1 teaspoon olive oil

8 drops lavender

2 drops geranium

2 drops carrot seed

Aromatherapy Facial Oil for Dry Skin #2

3/4 ounce apricot kernel oil

1/4 ounce avocado oil

1 teaspoon hazelnut oil

8 drops sandalwood

4 drops lavender

Aromatherapy Facial Oil For Sensitive Skin

1/2 ounce jojoba oil

1/2 ounce olive oil

2 drops rose

3 drops chamomile (Roman)

2 drops neroli

Aromatherapy Blemish Blend #1

5 drops tea tree

10 drops lavender

3 drops chamomile (Roman)

1 drop sandalwood

Mix essential oils into 3 ounces of aloe vera juice and 1 teaspoon witch hazel. Shake vigorously before applying to blemished areas.

Aromatherapy Blemish Blend #2

3 drops tea tree

3 drops geranium

4 drops lavender

1 drop chamomile (Roman)

1 drop juniper (berry)

Mix essential oils into 2 ounces of aloe vera juice and 1 teaspoon witch hazel. Shake vigorously before applying to blemished areas.

Aromatherapy Spot Blemish Blend

1 ounce aloe vera juice

1 teaspoon witch hazel

8 drops lavender

4 drops chamomile (Roman)

2 drops tea tree

1 drops juniper (berry)

1 drop geranium

Mix well and shake vigorously prior to use. Apply with a clean cotton swab directly on the blemish. This is a strong dilution, so it is not recommended for large areas.

Aromatherapy Facial Oil for Mature Skin #1

1/2 ounce jojoba oil

1/2 ounce sweet almond or canola oil

1 teaspoon olive oil

1/2 teaspoon flaxseed or borage oil

5 drops frankincense

3 drops neroli

5 drops lavender

Aromatherapy Facial Oil for Mature Skin #2

1/2ounce jojoba oil

1/2 ounce hazelnut oil

1 teaspoon squalene oil

contents of one capsule of vitamin E

8 drops lavender

2 drops frankincense

2 drops ylang ylang

2 drops carrot seed

Aromatherapy Facial Oil for Mature Skin #3

3/4 ounce avocado oil

1/4 ounce jojoba oil

1 teaspoon flaxseed or borage oil

5 drops frankincense

3 drops sandalwood

2 drops rose

2 drops lavender

Masks

to deep-cleanse, condition, and nourish

Masks are applied in a thick layer to a clean face. The neck can be included, if desired. Most masks should not be applied near the eyes. If the mask begins to dry out before the recommended time, mist it to keep it moist. While the mask is on, lie down with your feet slightly raised and cover the eyes with water-moistened eye pads.

Honey Mask *(for all skin types)*

This mask increases circulation to the skin and will smooth, soften, and moisturize.

To use: Warm 1 tablespoon of honey and apply to a clean face. Leave on for 15 minutes. Pat and press the honey to stimulate the skin. Rinse with warm water followed by a cool-water splash.

Clay Mask *(for all skin types except dry and mature)*

To make: Mix 1 rounded tablespoon of a good facial-quality clay (available at natural food stores) with enough water or milk to make a smooth paste. Add a few drops of olive oil (or any vegetable oil), a few drops of vinegar, and a spoonful of honey. If this mixture is too runny, add a little more clay. If it is too dry, add a little more water or milk.

To use: Apply to clean face and neck and leave on for 15 minutes. Rinse with warm water followed by a cool-water splash.

Simple Oatmeal Mask *(for all skin types)*

To make: Cook either instant oatmeal or rolled oats according to manufacturers' instructions. Allow to cool to a temperature that is slightly warm.

To use: Apply to clean skin and leave on for 15 minutes. Rinse with warm water followed by a cool-water splash.

Milk and Honey Mask *(for all skin types)*

To make: Mix 1 tablespoon honey and 1 tablespoon yogurt. Add powdered milk to thicken to a smooth paste.

To use: Apply to clean skin for 15 minutes. Rinse well with warm water followed by a cool-water splash.

Aromatherapy Clay Mask *(for normal skin)*

To make: Mix 1 tablespoon of facial-quality clay with 1 teaspoon of honey, 3 drops of essential oil of geranium, and enough aloe vera juice or water to make a paste.

To use: Apply to clean skin for 15 minutes. Rinse with warm water and follow with a cool-water splash.

Aromatherapy Clay/Oatmeal Mask *(for dry skin)*

To make: Mix 1 teaspoon of clay with 1 tablespoon of instant oatmeal or oat flour, 1 teaspoon honey, 1 teaspoon olive oil, and enough water to make a paste. Add 1 drop of essential oil of rose and 1 drop of essential oil of lavender.

To use: Apply to clean skin for 15 minutes. Rinse with warm water and follow with a cool-water splash.

Aromatherapy Clay/Witch Hazel Mask *(for oily skin)*

To make: Mix 1 tablespoon clay, 1 teaspoon aloe vera juice, 1 teaspoon witch hazel, and enough water to make a paste. Add 1 drop of essential oil of tea tree, 1 drop of essential oil of lavender, and 1 drop of essential oil of peppermint.

To use: Apply to clean skin for 15 minutes. Rinse with warm water and follow with a cool-water splash.

Aromatherapy Rejuvenating Mask *(for mature skin)*

To make: Mix 1 teaspoon of facial-quality clay, 1 teaspoon of instant oatmeal or oat flour, 1/2 tablespoon powdered milk, 1 teaspoon honey, 1 teaspoon avocado or olive oil, and enough water to make a paste. Add one drop of essential oil of frankincense and one drop of essential oil of neroli, lavender, or rose.

To use: Apply to clean skin for 10 minutes. Rinse with warm water and follow with a cool-water splash.

Carrot Mask *(for normal to dry skin)*

To make: Steam a large carrot well and then mash thoroughly, adding a little water if necessary to make a paste.

To use: Apply to clean skin for 10 minutes. Rinse with warm water and follow with a cool-water splash.

Apple Mask *(for normal to dry skin)*

To make: Thoroughly steam a peeled and cored apple. Mash and mix with a small amount of whole milk and honey.

To use: Apply to clean skin for 15 minutes. Rinse with warm water and follow with a cool-water splash.

Baking Soda Mask *(for blemished skin)*

To make: Mix 2 teaspoons of baking soda with water to form a paste.

To use: Apply to clean skin that is troubled with blemishes for 15 minutes. Rinse with cool water.

Clay Mask *(for blemished skin)*

To make: Mix 1 heaping tablespoon of facial clay with enough water to form a paste. Add 1 drop of essential oil of cypress, 1 drop of lavender, and 1 drop of chamomile (Roman).

To use: Apply to clean skin for 15 minutes. Rinse well with cool water.

Banana and Honey Mask *(for normal to dry skin)*

To make: Mash together 1/2 ripe banana with 1 teaspoon honey.

To use: Apply to clean skin for 15 minutes. Rinse with warm water and follow with a cool-water splash.

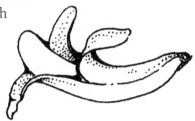

Facial Misters

to refresh and hydrate the skin

Herbal Facial Mister

To make: Steep 1 tablespoon of your favorite herb or blend of herbs in 1 cup of boiling water for 30 minutes. Strain and keep refrigerated. Replace every 4 days. For suggested herbal combinations, see "Herbal Cleansing Milk" at the beginning of this chapter.

Waters for Facial Misting

Mineral water

Aloe vera juice (must be the brand that has a water-like consistency)

True aromatherapy hydrosols (the water that is left after a plant has been distilled to remove the essential oils)

Eight ounces of pure water mixed with 10 drops of an essential oil or blend of essential oils. Shake vigorously before each use.

Massage Oils and Body Oils

to soothe, condition, and pamper

Basic Massage Oil

1 part avocado oil

2 parts sweet almond oil

1 part safflower oil

1/2 part jojoba oil

Herbal Massage Oil

#1 Infuse your favorite blend of herbs in the basic massage oil by putting in a glass container 1/4 cup of dried herbs and 1 cup of oil. Place the container in the sun or a warm location for 5-10 days. Shake daily and then strain and bottle.

#2 Add herbal extracts to the basic massage oil. Use a total of 50 drops of an herbal extract or blend of herbal extracts to every cup of oil.

Massage Oil *(for the hands)*

1 teaspoon wheat germ oil

400 I.U. vitamin E

2 oz. avocado oil

2 oz. apricot kernel oil

4 drops of essential oil of lemon

Massage Oil to Cool the Feet

1 teaspoon wheat germ oil

1 tablespoon olive oil

2 tablespoons canola oil

3 drops of essential oil of peppermint or rosemary

Aromatherapy Energizing Body Oil #1

4 ounces of canola or sweet almond oil (or Basic Massage Oil)

15 drops rosemary

5 drops geranium

10 drops clary sage

10 drops lavender

2 drops peppermint

5 drops grapefruit

3 drops basil

Aromatherapy Energizing Body Oil #2

4 ounces of canola or sweet almond oil (or Basic Massage Oil)

10 drops peppermint

13 drops rosemary

8 drops grapefruit

8 drops orange

Energizing Body Oil #3

4 ounces canola or sweet almond oil (or Basic Massage Oil)

30 drops rosemary

10 drops juniper (berry)

6 drops peppermint

Relaxing Body Oil #1

4 ounces of canola or sweet almond oil (or Basic Massage Oil)

20 drops lavender

5 drops marjoram

5 drops bergamot

5 drops chamomile (Roman)

2 drops ylang ylang

10 drops orange

3 drops geranium

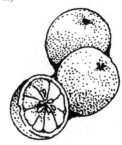

Relaxing Body Oil #2

4 ounces of canola or sweet almond oil (or Basic Massage Oil)

20 drops sandalwood

15 drops chamomile (Roman)

5 drops rose

5 drops rosewood

Relaxing Body Oil #3

4 ounces of canola or sweet almond oil (or Basic Massage Oil)
15 drops chamomile (Roman)
15 drops clary sage
15 drops lavender

Relaxing Body Oil #4

4 ounces of canola or sweet almond oil (or Basic Massage Oil)
15 drops ylang ylang
15 drops cedarwood
5 drops clary sage
5 drops lavender
5 drops chamomile (Roman)

Sore Muscle Body Oil

4 ounces of canola or sweet almond oil (or Basic Massage Oil)
15 drops eucalyptus
15 drops rosemary
10 drops lavender
5 drops marjoram

PART II

Natural
Skin Care

Alternative
Techniques

8

Acupressure

*The healing touch of acupressure reduces tension,
increases circulation and enables the body to relax
deeply. By relieving stress, acupressure strengthens
resistance to disease and promotes wellness.*
 —Michael Reed Gach,
  Acupressure's Potent Points

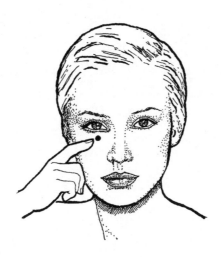

For Health & Well Being

A cupressure is part of a 5,000-year-old Oriental medical philosophy and practice that focuses on preventing disease and maintaining good health. This philosophy recognizes the body's miraculous power to regenerate and repair itself. Acupressure uses the fingers to press key points on the body and is aimed at restoring the body's intricate balance, thus helping it to heal itself and creating a natural pathway to good health. Acupressure is used today as a solo treatment as well as an adjunct to other medical modalities. It has been used successfully to treat a variety of physical problems such as headaches, muscular pain, sports injuries, and backaches. Because it releases accumulated tension, acupressure can help psychological problems that result from repressed emotions and stress.

Central to understanding acupressure is the concept of *chi*. According to Oriental medicine, *chi* is the absolute basis for all forms of life in the universe. It is the Chinese term for "life sustaining energy." Imbalance of the *chi*—either too much or too little—is believed to be the root of all illness. When *chi* is gone, life is gone. Oriental medicine aims to strengthen, balance and harmonize the *chi*, and acupressure is one technique for accomplishing this goal.

The points on the skin used in acupressure are specific places that easily transmit bioelectrical impulses in the body. When a point is pressed, it releases muscle tension caused by stress in the body, brings about relaxation and restores the flow of energy. This allows an increase of blood flow and oxygen supply. Toxins are released and carried away. This process helps to increase the body's vital energy and its ability to resist disease. It is effective whether it is done by one person to another or done on oneself.

❧ *For Skin Care*

Acupressure is an effective way to enhance beauty and vitality and the techniques compliment your natural skin care program. The skin responds particularly well to acupressure. Practiced regularly, the techniques can improve the condition of the complexion, tone and relax the facial muscles, bring vitality to the skin, and help reduce the signs of aging. It can help balance glandular activity, nourish the skin and underlying structures, calm the nerves, and strengthen the muscle fibers.

Simple and effective, the following four exercises can become part of your daily skin care routine. Choose to do all of them or the ones you enjoy the most. Use the balls of the fingertips or palms of the hands to apply pressure to the key points, usually on both sides of the face (bi-laterally). The technique for applying the pressure is firm yet gentle. The sensation should be slightly uncomfortable while still feeling good.

As you begin to use acupressure, you will discover that some points are very sensitive. This is a good indication that you are correctly positioned on that point. The point will become less sensitive the more often it is pressed. Do not press any point if it is extremely painful. As acupressure's effects are powerful yet subtle, it should be practiced every day, on a regular schedule to be the most effective.

1

In China, women regularly practice skin revitalizing techniques. It is believed that a wrinkle is caused by stagnation of the body's energy (*chi*). Stimulation to disperse the stagnation is achieved by acupressure as well as light massage.

The following technique tones the entire eye area and helps to prevent and eliminate crow's feet. Using the middle finger of each hand, massage around each eye simultaneously, following the direction of the arrows in Figure 1. Apply a small amount of moisturizer or massage oil, and use slight pressure as you glide over the eyebrow and underneath the eye, along the bone. Circle the eye thirty times and practice this once a day.

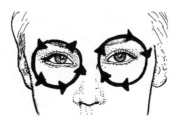

Figure 1

2

Stimulating the points in Figure 2 revitalize the eye area and can prevent and soften fine lines and wrinkles around the eyes. Press each point for three seconds, release for a moment, and repeat for thirty counts. (This method of applying pressure has a stimulating effect as opposed to prolonged pressure which has a more relaxing effect). This should be practiced three times a day.

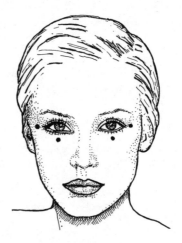

Figure 2

3

"Big Washing Face Massage" is a favorite Oriental skin care technique, and was taught to the author by Yen Wei Choong, an acupuncturist in Northern California. It is used to tone and stimulate the entire face, clear the complexion, and prevent wrinkles. To begin, wash and dry your hands. Then, with your palms together, rub your hands back and forth rapidly (you will feel warmth) thirty-six times. This puts "*chi* on the palm," as Yen Wei described. Next, move your hands over your face in an upward motion, covering the entire face including your ears. Your hands gently touch the skin, without pulling. Each hand moves in a circle beginning at the chin, moving up alongside the nose, over the eyes to the forehead, along the hairline, over the ears, and back to the chin again. The circular motion should be completed thirty-six times. Yen Wei suggests doing this every day as part of your skin care routine. "It will harmonize the *chi* of the face, protecting against all facial imbalances, including wrinkling, blemishes, or sallow coloring."

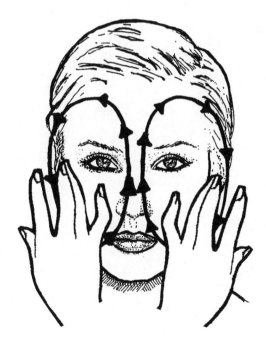

Figure 3

4

The points in Figure 4 illustrate a full facial treatment designed to bring vitality to the complexion. This technique will smooth, tone, and help prevent wrinkles. Wash your hands and face. Using the index fingers, press each point indicated (most are bi-lateral), for five seconds. Then, tap the same point five times. Press them in the order they are numbered, beginning at the chin and working up toward the forehead.

For more information about acupressure and the complexion, see Chapter 4, "Alternative Techniques for Blemished Skin."

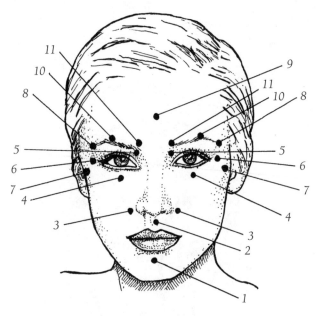

Figure 4

Recommended Reading

Acupressure's Potent Points, Michael Reed Gach (New York: Bantam Books, 1990).
New Beauty: Acupressure Face Lift, Lindsey Wagner & Robert Klein (Englewood Cliffs, NJ: Prentice Hall, 1987).

9

Aromatherapy

Aromatherapy nourishes our bodies, minds and spirits in a vital, restorative way. Its benefits inspire celebration of our own essence and its unique rhythm with nature.
—Alexandra Avery, Aromatherapist

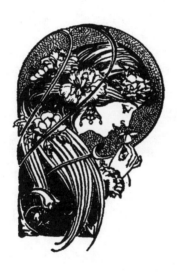

For Health & Well Being

Aromatherapy uses the essential oils from aromatic plants for the purpose of restoring or enhancing health and beauty. It is being used today in the fields of medicine, psychology, and cosmetology and has been acknowledged as a viable method of treatment.

Essential oils have been used for hundreds of years by a variety of cultures for both medicinal and religious purposes. Aromatic oils, as they are also called, were used in China, by the Greeks and the Romans. They were eventually brought to England with the earliest written record of their use there in the 13th century. In 1652, Nicholas Culpeper wrote a book on the medicinal properties of plants and their essential oils. However, by the 19th century, chemists endeavored to produce chemical copies of the fragrance of essential oils. These synthetic fragrances were much cheaper to produce but they lacked the medicinal properties of true essential oils, so they were useful only as perfumes. Scientists challenged to chemically reproduce these elusive medicinal qualities then began to isolate the "active" ingredients and in many cases were successful. The "modern" world of scientific medicine—then just emerging—lost interest in plants for therapeutic value, and at this point, their wide use was curtailed in the West. But in the 20th century, a renewed interest in natural products and treatments emerged. In the 1930s, Renée Gattefossé, a French chemist, coined the term "aromatherapy." He is considered to be the father of modern aromatherapy and wrote the first book on the subject.

The essential oils used in aromatherapy are extracted from many parts of the aromatic plant: the leaves, stems, flowers, seeds, roots, barks, woods, fruits, and resins. The scent of the plant is due to the essential oil content. The oils are a concentrated form of plant energy possessing the qualities inherent in that particular plant, and many times more potent than comparable dried herbs. Plants used for aromatherapy oils must be picked at certain times of the day and year and in certain weather conditions. This is because the essential oil changes its chemical composition and moves from one part of the plant to another according to external influences. The most common method of extraction is distillation, but other methods such as enfleurage and cold expression are also used. True essential oils cannot be synthetically duplicated to perfection and are, indeed, one of nature's very special gifts.

Essential oils are not greasy. To demonstrate this, compare a pure, undiluted essential oil to a vegetable oil such as olive oil. Put a few drops of the essential oil on a piece of paper. Put a few drops of the vegetable oil near it. Check the two spots in a couple of hours. The essential oil will leave no mark but the vegetable oil will. This is due to the full evaporation of the essential oil and is why essential oils are also known as "etheric oils" due to their light, airy, and delicate nature.

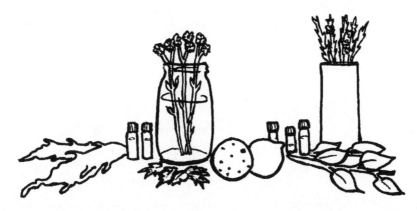

Examples of Plant Parts and Derived Essential Oil

Leaves & Stems:	Rosemary, geranium, marjoram, peppermint, clary sage, tea tree
Flowers:	Rose, ylang ylang, lavender, chamomile, jasmine, neroli
Seeds:	Carrot, nutmeg, coriander
Roots:	Ginger, vetivert
Barks:	Cinnamon, birch
Woods:	Sandalwood, cedarwood, rosewood
Fruits:	Orange, lemon, bergamot, tangerine, grapefruit
Resins:	Frankincense, myrrh

Essential oils used for aromatherapy purposes must be of high quality in order to be effective. The price of these oils will vary depending on the plant's availability, the amount of essential oil in the plant, and the exact method of distillation. Prices will also vary from season to season, depending on the success of the crop. Common plants that produce a great deal of essential oil can be relatively inexpensive. Plants that produce very little essential oil can be very, very expensive. Rose is one of the most expensive oils because it takes 2000 pounds of rose petals to produce one pound of essential rose oil.

Though essential oils can be expensive for the quantity, they are highly concentrated, so only a small amount is needed. Purchasing aromatherapy-grade essential oils for cosmetic use is an investment in quality and well worth the cost. (To protect your investment and slow the loss of potency, essential oils should be stored in a cool, dark place in a dark, glass bottle with a solid cap).

For Skin Care & the Psyche

Aromatherapy and the cosmetic use of essential oils have made a tremendous contribution to skin care. Every type of skin (such as oily, dry, and normal) can benefit. There are seven important properties that essential oils offer for care of the skin:

1. reduces pain
2. reduces inflammation
3. inhibits bacteria growth (nearly all essential oils are good antiseptics)
4. contracts the skin tissue
5. stimulates cell renewal
6. contracts small blood vessels
7. aids healing of wounds

In addition to reaping the marvelous benefits of aromatherapy for the skin, the user also benefits from the psychological effects. Essential oils affect us psychologically through our sense of smell. This process begins when the aroma enters the nose. Here, the air is warmed and filtered. When the aroma reaches the olfactory receptor sites, it "fits" onto the hairs there and triggers an enzyme reaction which, in turn, creates another reaction that goes to the olfactory bulb and sends information to the limbic system of the brain which receives and stores information experienced via our senses. This part of the brain is the site for much of our creativity, processing memory, emotions, and basic drives such as hunger. It is believed that here, in this very sensitive storehouse, essential oils affect how we feel.

Throughout the vast array of essential oils available from the plant world, a few stand out for their multiple applications and effectiveness in skin care. Listed below are the most popular cosmetic essential oils and their psychological benefits. (The latter is in italics.)

Popular Cosmetic Essential Oils

Carrot seed is especially good for dry, mature, or aging skins because it stimulates cell renewal and sebaceous gland activity in the skin. It is known as a rejuvenating oil and protects against skin damage due to weather exposure. It has a woody, earthy scent. *Carrot seed does not have qualities that are commonly used to benefit the psyche.*

Cedarwood has an astringent quality and helps to balance excessive oil secretion. It is good for oily, blemished, or congested skin and has a soft, woodsy fragrance. *Cedarwood calms anxiety and nervous tension while providing comfort and strength.*

Chamomile (Roman) is soothing, calming, and an anti-inflammatory. It is an analgesic (pain reducer) and disinfectant with a gentle nature. Chamomile is very good for dry, sensitive skin and because it has the ability to shrink small blood vessels, it can help reduce redness from enlarged capillaries that sensitive skin can be prone to. It is also good for calming allergic reaction. It has a light, sweet apple-like aroma. *Chamomile relieves depression, irritability, and insomnia, and calms the nerves.*

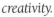**Clary sage** helps to promote the regeneration of skin cells and reduce inflammation. It is effective for dry and mature skin as well as blemished. It has a fresh, sweet, warm aroma. *Clary sage relaxes, relieves tension, and promotes emotional balance. It is an anti-depressant and inspires creativity.*

Frankincense is an excellent oil for mature skin because of its rejuvenating properties. It is used to reduce existing wrinkles and to deter their formation. It has a slight astringent action and promotes healing. It has a deep, woody, slightly spicy fragrance. *Frankincense is calming to the emotions and encourages a sense of belonging.*

Geranium is astringent, antiseptic, and it promotes speedy healing. It is excellent in balancing oil production, so it is well suited for all skin types, especially combination. It has deodorizing and cleansing qualities and stimulates the lymphatic system. Its fragrance is sweet and rich. *Geranium has anti-depressant, uplifting, and calming effects on the psyche.*

Jasmine can be used for all types of skin. Though it is a very expensive essential oil, only a small amount is needed. It has a toning, antiseptic quality, and is very soothing for dry, sensitive skin. It has a sweet, floral, exotic fragrance. *Jasmine relaxes the mind and helps to alleviate anger, nervousness, and worries.*

Lavender is considered to be the most useful and versatile of all the essential oils and is invaluable for all types of skin, including mature. It is soothing, antiseptic, anti-inflammatory, regenerative, and balancing. Lavender is one of the few oils that can be applied undiluted (neat) to the skin, and few people are allergic to it. It is excellent for the treatment of acne because it inhibits bacteria, soothes the skin, helps to balance overactive sebaceous glands, and reduces scarring by stimulating the growth of healthy new cells. It has a light, clear, full floral fragrance. *Lavender is soothing and uplifting to the psyche and relaxes the nervous system.*

 Lemon has the ability to stimulate white corpuscles that defend the body against infection. It is a powerful bactericide, an astringent, and a mild bleaching agent. Lemon oil can be irritating to the skin so it must be used in very low dilution and should be avoided by very sensitive skins. However, used as a facial wash, it is excellent for broken capillaries and greasy skin. It's fresh, clean scent appeals to almost everyone. *Lemon has uplifting, anti-depressant qualities.*

 Neroli is a gentle oil known for its rejuvenating qualities and is especially good for dry and mature skin. It stimulates new cell growth and may delay the deterioration of the connective tissues as they age. It is an expensive oil with a sweet, floral aroma. *Neroli calms the psyche and has aphrodisiac qualities.*

 Patchouli regenerates skin cells, calms inflammation, and helps to balance oil production. It is used for dry, mature, and blemished skin and has a powerful distinctive fragrance that is heavy, earthy, and woody as well as sweet, spicy and exotic. *Patchouli is an anti-depressant, relieves anxiety, and reduces mental fatigue.*

 Rose is considered the "queen" of essential oils. It is good for all types of skin but especially dry, sensitive, or aging. It is an excellent antiseptic and anti-inflammatory agent. Rose can help reduce the redness of enlarged capillaries when used regularly. Its fragrance is a deep, sweet floral that has been treasured through the ages. *Rose is a gentle yet powerful anti-depressant. It soothes the nerves and is renowned for its aphrodisiac qualities.*

 Rosemary is used in skin care for its astringent, stimulating, and strong antiseptic qualities. It can benefit most types of skin, depending on the concentration. It is especially good for dry and mature skin when increased circulation is desirable. It also stimulates skin metabolism and lymph drainage. It has a strong, clear, warm herbal fragrance. *Rosemary helps to eliminate mental fatigue and is said to improve the ability to concentrate and think clearly.*

Rosewood stimulates new cell growth, helps to balance oil secretions, and soothes the skin. It is used for all types and skin and has a soft, sweet, woodsy fragrance. *Rosewood is an antidepressant, relieves stress, and strengthens the nervous system.*

Sandalwood is good for all types of skin. It is soothing, inhibits bacterial growth, and is slightly astringent. Its fragrance is deep and warm, woody and exotic. *Sandalwood is comforting and relaxing and has aphrodisiac qualities.*

Tea Tree is an especially powerful antiseptic that is active against bacteria, fungus, and viruses. It is also a strong immune system stimulant. It can irritate the skin so care must be taken to dilute the oil when using it on sensitive skin. It is excellent as a wash for acne, and a small drop can be applied undiluted on pimples to help clear them quickly. Its fragrance is fresh, medicinal, and pungent. *Tea tree does not have qualities that are commonly used to benefit the psyche.*

Ylang ylang is suitable for all skin types because it has a balancing effect on the sebaceous glands. It moisturizes, softens, and rejuvenates. It has a heavy, very sweet floral aroma. *Ylang ylang is soothing, and counteracts anger and frustration. It is an anti-depressant, an aphrodisiac, and a euphoric.*

Practical Applications in Skin Care

Essential oils can be used at home in masks, massage oils, and facial oils. They can also be used in compresses, facial misters and washes as a part of your daily skin care routine. Essential oils can be added to commercial moisturizers, cleansers, or toners to enhance the products' effectiveness.

Masks

Essential oils are easily added to any mask base such as clay, yogurt, or mashed fruits or vegetables. Use four drops of an essential oil or essential oil blend. If you have very sensitive skin, use fewer drops and only the most gentle essential oils such as chamomile or rose. See Chapter 3 for details about using masks.

Massage Oils

Massage oils are used on the whole body (except the face) and are designed to provide "slip" to the skin so the hands glide smoothly. An aromatherapy massage oil is made of essential oils diluted in a base oil (also called carrier oil). Together, they enhance the physical manipulation of massage by providing beneficial botanical properties from the essential oils and emolliency and protection from the base oils. The general recipe for making an aromatherapy massage oil is to use an approximate 2 percent solution or 25 drops of essential oil in 2 ounces of base oil. Shake well. (Recipes for massage oils are given in Chapter 7, "Making Your Own Skin Care Products.")

NOTE: Though 2 percent is appropriate for a general guideline, this could vary depending on the essential oil, the intended use of the massage oil, and the type of skin on which it is used. Sensitive skin may require a 1 percent solution.

Facial Oils

Facial oils are formulated similarly to massage oils but they are designed specifically for the face. They usually contain the finest and most expensive essential oils—ones that would be too costly to use all over the body. In addition, the base oil is a blend of oils that are especially nurturing to the facial skin such as jojoba, kukui, hazelnut, or squalene. As a guideline, use 20 drops of your chosen essential oil or blend of essential oils to 2 ounces of base oil. For sensitive skin use 10 drops.

Compresses

Compresses (folded cloths) can be used cosmetically on the face with either cool water to contract the skin for a bracing effect, or warm water to relax it. Washcloths or cloth diapers make excellent compresses. Essential oils can be added straight into a basin or bowl of water for compresses, but because oil and water do not mix, it is best if the essential oil is first added to a dispersing agent to evenly distribute it in the water. This prevents 'hot spots' of the essential oil that may irritate the skin. Essential oils of lavender, neroli, or rose are good for all skin types. Add two to five drops of essential oil to a small amount (1 teaspoon) of vinegar or vodka for dispersing, and then add this to the water in which the compress is dipped. Stir well and immerse the cloth. Wring well and apply it to the skin.

Facial Misters

Add 5 to 10 drops of essential oil or blend of essential oils for every 8 ounces of water in your pump sprayer. Remember that essential oils and water do not mix, so shake vigorously before misting the skin. Be careful not to get this mist in the eyes because it could cause irritation. See Chapter 3 for more on facial misting.

Facial Wash

A facial wash is similar to a toner but designed with a more specific purpose such as a tea tree oil wash for blemished skin or a chamomile wash for inflamed skin. A facial wash is made by mixing 5 to 10 drops of essential oil in 1 cup of pure water. Shake vigorously, dampen a cotton ball and wipe the skin. Lemon oil is good for broken capillaries and greasy, congested skin. Lavender, rose, chamomile, rosewood, and geranium are good for all types of skin.

Add to Products

Essential oils blend well and are very effective when added to creams, lotions, moisturizers, or any product that contains oil. Essential oils can also be added to toners, aftershaves and masks. In these cases, it is recommended that you start with a simple, *unscented* product and follow this guideline: 20-25 drops to 2 ounces of product.

The Safety of Essential Oils

As with any active, therapeutic substance, essential oil use may become a safety concern. Because essential oils are pharmacologically effective, they can be harmful to the body if used incorrectly. Chronic toxicity can result when a small amount of a potentially hazardous oil is applied repeatedly to the skin over a long period of time. Gradual kidney or liver damage could occur. Some oils have been known to cause abortion. However, Robert Tisserand, author of *The Safety Data Manual* for essential oils, explains that toxicity can be tackled by completely avoiding the essential oils which present a risk. Many aromatherapy books will provide you with a list of these oils.

Aside from toxic reactions, there can also be irritation and allergic reactions. Skin irritation can occur with almost any essential oil because they are so concentrated. This problem is easily solved by properly diluting the oil. The more the oil is diluted, the less irritating it becomes. Allergic reactions are a risk when using essential oils, though they are not common. However, diluting the oil will not prevent this problem. Allergic reaction most often occurs in people with sensitive skin. Though they will not react to all essential oils, care must be taken in oil selection as well as in the dilution.

Anyone preparing to use or work with essential oils would be well-advised to study one or more of the many books now available in order to understand the subtleties and counter-indications of using essential oils.

Recommended Reading

The Aromatherapy Book: Applications and Inhalations, Jeanne Rose (Berkeley, CA: North Atlantic Books, 1992).

Aromatherapy An A-Z , Patricia Davis (England: C.W. Daniel Company Limited, 1988).

The Complete Book of Essential Oils & Aromatherapy, Valerie Ann Worwood (San Rafael, CA: New World Library, 1991).

Aromatherapy: Answers to the Most Commonly Asked Questions, Michael Scholes (Los Angeles, CA: Aromatherapy Seminars, 1993).

10

Ayurveda

---

*Ayurveda gives us the direction to eat, breathe
and think properly for the blossoming of internal
radiance that is ageless beauty.*
  —*Pratima Raichur, Botanist &
    Ayurvedic Skin Care Specialist*

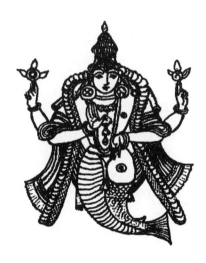

For Health & Well-Being

Ayurveda, which means "life knowledge," is the art of healing and rejuvenation, and has been used in India for thousands of years. Ayurveda has the distinction of being the "oldest medical system known to man and the oldest and most comprehensive spiritual teachings in the world."[1] Ayurveda is unique in that it thoroughly encompasses and nurtures the mind, body, and spirit of the human being. It holds that a person can create balance in their internal forces by altering their diet and habits of living to counteract conditions in the external environment. The practical guidelines that Ayurveda offers for daily living increase energy and creativity, and empower the individual to live a harmonious life.

According to Ayurveda, everyone is born with a genetically determined, basic constitution. These constitutional types are expressions of the five elements that describe the qualities of energy as it is displayed in the universe. They are ether (space), air, fire, water, and earth. These five elements form three basic constitutions in the human body known as *Vata* (ether and air), *Pitta* (fire and water) and *Kapha* (water and earth). Identifying your constitutional type *(dosha)* helps to establish your guidelines for healthy living. Everyone is a combination of all three types with one or two being dominate. It remains the same from birth. The goal is to work with the basic constitution to balance all five elements. Imbalance, according to Ayurveda, is what causes discomfort, disease and premature aging.

As you read through the doshas to determine your own, remember there is no value judgment of "good" or "bad" placed on these characteristics. Most people are a combination of two dominant doshas. You will be able to relate to certain parts of each dosha, but *your* dosha (or doshas) will be the one that best describes you.

The Doshas

Vata

Vata controls movement in the body.

Vata people are what we might call "airy" people and they can be unpredictable. They are creative, active, alert, and restless. They move about quickly, speak quickly, and do things quickly. They also tire quickly.

Physically, they are usually small-boned with thin, under-developed frames. They may be underweight. Veins and muscles are visible, and their hair and skin tend to be dry. Their fingernails are rough and brittle. There is a tendency to perspire less than the other types. Vata people sleep lightly, and their hands and feet are often cold. They usually prefer foods that are sweet, sour, and salty.

Psychologically, Vata types tend to hold fear and are over-stressed and nervous. Such people may be emotionally unstable. They have a short memory but are quick to understanding a situation. They tend to be impatient and lack assertiveness and confidence.

Vata skin is pale, cool, and often dehydrated, with a "cracked" appearance due to the "dry" aspect of the Vata nature. Often there are circles under the eyes, premature wrinkling, and a tendency towards moles.

Pitta

Pitta controls metabolism and digestion in the body.

Pitta people have a "fiery" nature with average strength and endurance. They are very intelligent, with good powers of concentration and ability to speak in public. They are witty and outspoken but may be argumentative.

Physically, they are of moderate weight, height, and muscle development. There is a tendency to perspire heavily, and the hands and feet are warm. The hair is thin and silky with a tendency towards premature greying and balding. The fingernails are soft. Pitta people have a strong metabolism and appetite with good digestion. They usually like foods that are sweet, bitter, and astringent. They sleep well for a moderate amount of time. They do not tolerate sunlight or heat well.

Psychologically, Pitta types are ambitious and like to be leaders. They tend to feel anger, hate, frustration, and jealousy more than the other types.

The Pitta skin is soft, reddish, yellowish, or fair. It can be sensitive and dehydrated. There is a tendency toward broken capillaries, rashes, itching, eruptions, allergic reactions, and freckles. There is less of a tendency to wrinkling than for Vata.

Kapha

Kapha controls the structure of the body.

The Kapha person is generally healthy, happy, and peaceful. They are our relaxed, "earthy" folks. This type tends to have a thick frame, well-developed bodies and may have a tendency to be overweight. They have great strength, endurance and stamina. Kapha people speak slower and move slower than average. Their hair is thick, soft, and often wavy. They have a regular appetite and digest slowly. They may prefer foods that are pungent, bitter, and astringent. They perspire moderately and sleep well for extended periods.

Psychologically, kapha people tend to be affectionate, tolerant, calm, forgiving, and loving. However, they also have a tendency towards greed, envy, and possessiveness. They can be slow to understand things but once they do, the information is retained well.

The Kapha skin is lustrous due to a high oil content but has a tendency toward blemish problems. It has a soft, pale, and cool quality to it.

The Diet

Ayurveda offers general diet guidelines as well as specific guidelines for each constitutional type. The appropriate diet is considered critical to good health as well as a beautiful complexion. Generally, it is recommended to eat at regular, established meal times. Eat in a peaceful setting without distractions and never when you are emotionally upset or in a hurry because it impairs digestion. Eat foods in season and try to avoid foods that are of diminished "life force" such as canned or frozen. Chew your food well (32 times is recommended) and eat at a slow to moderate pace. No more than the equivalent of two handfuls of food should be eaten at any one time. Overeating results in poor digestion and stresses the digestive tract. Sipping room temperature water during a meal is recommended to aid digestion, though large amounts of water after a meal should be avoided, because it impairs the digestion.

All constitutional types must avoid excessive amounts of refined foods such as sugar and white flour products. Alcohol, fried foods, caffeine, red meats, hard cheeses, salt, iced drinks, and raw foods should also be limited. (Raw foods are only used periodically for "cleansing" purposes.) Whole grains and whole grain products, beans, fresh fruits and steamed vegetables, warm or cool drinks (not hot or cold), and water are recommended.

The specific guidelines for each dosha are designed to balance your constitutional type. For example, if you have lots of "fire", you would want to avoid "fiery" foods such as chilies, garlic, or onion. It would be best to cool and balance the fire with watery foods such as celery or cucumber.

If you are of a Vata constitution, focus on a diet that balances your basic "airy" nature. Cooked vegetables are good for you but raw vegetables should be avoided. Gas-producing vegetables such as broccoli, cauliflower, brussel sprouts, and cabbage are not good. Most varieties of sweet fruits are fine but avoid apples, pears, and dried fruits. All dairy products in moderation are acceptable as well as all oils. Any sweetener can be used except white sugar. All spices are good. All nuts and seeds are fine in moderation, and the best grains are rice, wheat, and oats. Beef and poultry can be eaten but lamb and pork should not. Vata people should drink eight glasses of water a day.

If you are of a Pitta dosha, you are balancing "water" and "fire." Avoid pungent vegetables such as beets, carrots, and eggplant. Sweet and bitter vegetables such as asparagus, broccoli, and brussel sprouts are good. Sweet fruits such as apples, oranges, pears, and figs are good but sour fruits such as grapefruit and cranberries are not. Barley, oats, rice (white or basmati), and wheat are the grains for the Pitta person. The best meat is white poultry. The white of eggs is also acceptable. Nuts and seeds should be avoided except coconut, sunflower, and pumpkin. All sweeteners are good except molasses and honey. Most spices should be avoided except coriander and cumin. Coconut, olive, sunflower, and soy oils are good and dairy products such as butter, ghee (clarified butter), cottage cheese, and milk can be used. Do not use soured dairy products. Pitta people should drink six to seven glasses of water a day.

The Kapha dosha needs to balance the water and earth elements. Avoid sweet and juicy vegetables. Pungent and bitter vegetables such as asparagus, beets, and broccoli are recommended. Avoid sweet and sour fruits. Acceptable are apples, apricots, berries, pears, and prunes. The best grains are barley, corn, millet, and basmati rice. Brown rice and wheat should be avoided. Chicken, turkey, and eggs are fine. Use no sweeteners except raw honey. Use no nuts at all and no seeds except sunflower and pumpkin. All spices can be used except salt. Use no dairy except ghee and goat milk. Use almond, corn, or sunflower oil and only in small quantities. Kapha people do well drinking five to six glasses of water a day.

Breathing

Ayurveda views correct breathing as a very important part of healthy living. The breath is the manifestation of energy in the body, and if you control your breath, you control your life force. Ayurveda suggests that we are given, at birth, a certain number of breaths. Controlling the breath is recommended so as not to "use up" our allotted amount too soon.

Breathing exercises in Ayurveda are called "pranayama" and are designed to balance the consciousness. Ayurvedic thought holds that when one is practicing pranayama, one experiences the true meaning of peace and love. There are different breathing exercises for each constitution. The Vata dosha should practice alternate breathing—in left, out right, in right, out left. (Use the middle finger and thumb to block the appropriate nostril). The Pitta dosha should breathe in the left nostril and out the right. The Kapha dosha breathes in the right and out the left. In all cases, breathe in to the count of four and out to the count of four. Slowly fill the abdomen with air first, then the stomach, the lower lungs, and lastly, the upper lung. (Of course, only the lungs actually fill with air.) To exhale, empty the abdomen first, then stomach, then lungs. It is suggested that you do your breathing exercise upon arising in the morning for three to five minutes.

Thought

An important part of Ayurveda, meditation is practiced to gain control of the emotions, mastery over thoughts, and to bring awareness, harmony, and order to daily living. Making available a very deep well of resources, meditation awakens intelligence and creativity and reduces the effects of stress.

Practiced regularly, meditation can help alleviate the symptoms of negative emotions, which according to Ayurveda, can adversely affect the functioning of a particular part of the body and, in turn, affect the skin. Vata people tend to hold on to fear, which affects the kidneys, resulting in dehydrated skin and puffiness and discoloration around the eyes. Pitta types suppress the emotions, which affects the liver and changes the flora in the small intestines, resulting in hives, rashes, and broken capillaries. The possessiveness and attachment of Kapha people affects their lungs, which results in respiratory and sinus problems as well as acne and excessive skin oiliness.

NOTE: In order to learn meditation and pranayama correctly, it is advised that one learn from an instructor of Ayurveda or yoga.

For Skin Care

The principles of Ayurveda are the foundation for a wholistic and natural approach to skin care. The complexion, after all, is a reflection of our mental and physical well-being. Ayurveda works with whole-food nutrition, proper breathing, meditation, herbs, and essential oils to achieve balance that reflects in healthy, beautiful skin. Ayurveda teaches us that real beauty is health—physically, mentally, and spiritually—and it is a reflection from within. Taking care to eat, breathe, and think well offers the rewards of ageless beauty.

Because we are affected by what contacts our skin (through absorption) and by scents we receive through our nose (aromatherapy), care must be taken that cosmetics are in tune with the constitution and have basic properties that support health and well-being. For these reasons, Ayurvedic skin care employs only natural substances to cleanse, condition, and moisturize.

Ayurveda dictates that the skin be cleansed gently without harsh soaps or detergents to leave natural protective oils intact. To cleanse the face and body, the basic format of massaging first with a small amount of oil suited to your constitution is recommended. Vata people can use sesame or apricot oil. Pitta can use coconut or sunflower, and Kapha should use olive or canola.[2] After a thorough, gentle massage, use a small amount of chick pea or rice flour and continue massaging to absorb the excess oil and loosened soil. The skin is then rinsed well with warm water and splashed with cool. To complete the cleansing process, the face should be steamed for five minutes. If this is not convenient, you may use facial compresses instead. (See Chapter 3, "Compresses.") Both the steaming and the compresses serve two purposes—they hydrate and cleanse the skin.

After cleansing, a blend of essential oils is applied to condition the skin and prevent moisture loss. For the Vata constitution, use essential oils that will be warming such as vetivert or camphor combined in a one-to-one ratio with "grounding" oils such as rose or sandalwood. Pitta people need essential oils that will cool and calm such as rose or sandalwood. Kapha people should use essential oils that stimulate and warm such as myrrh, ashvagandha, or neem. To make your conditioning facial oil, use twenty to twenty-five drops of essential oil to two ounces of base oil. (For each constitution, the base oil can be the same that is used for cleansing.)

When the facial blends are used regularly with "marma point" massage (similar to acupressure), they will soften the skin and reduce the visible signs of aging. You can use the marma points as illustrated below, once a day, after applying the facial blend. Vata should use a light pressure; Pitta should alternate light and heavy pressure; and Kapha needs deep pressure. Press each point once for fifteen seconds.

Common skin problems can be eliminated by a balanced Ayurvedic skin care program, but when problems do arise, an Ayurvedic point of view helps to

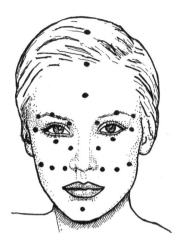

marma points

explain the causes and effects. Chapped lips are a Vata condition that can be caused by a dry colon. Internally and externally, dry, cold conditions must be avoided. A light film of sesame oil will help prevent moisture loss. Warm, wet, and cooked foods are recommended. Wrinkles in any culture are primarily a result of weather exposure; this is a dry (Vata) condition. The skin should be well hydrated *internally* and well lubricated and protected *externally*. Ayurveda also recommends massage as one of the best ways to prevent wrinkles. In a lying-down position, for three to five minutes a day, gently massage the face with warmed sesame oil, beginning with the forehead and proceeding to the temples, the nose, the cheeks, and then the chin and neck. Do not pull excessively on the skin, but concentrate on stimulating the underlying tissues.

(For more information about Ayurvedic skin care, contact Janaki at the American Association of Ayurvedic Aesthetics, P.O. Box 5121, Berkeley, CA 94705).

Recommended Reading

Ayurveda: The Science of Self-Healing, Dr. Vasant Lad (Santa Fe, NM: Lotus Press, 1984).

The Yoga of Herbs: An Ayurvedic Guide to Herbal Medicine, Dr. David Frawley and Dr. Vasant Lad (Santa Fe, NM: Lotus Press, 1986).

11

Color Therapy

Color can transform our environment and increase our productivity. It can enhance our social life, and improve our state of health. It can be used to develop our self-awareness and make us more fully alive and more colorful human beings.
—Howard and Dorothy Sun, Color Therapists

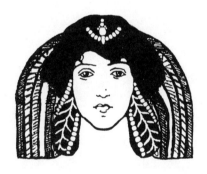

For Health & Well-Being

Color therapy uses colors and light to beneficially affect our physical, emotional, and spiritual well-being. Color therapy has been used through the ages and is believed to have its roots in ancient Egypt and Greece, where color temples were built. The temples had seven compartments—each containing one of the colors of the rainbow. When people visited, they were put into the colored compartment that would benefit them the most.[1]

Hippocrates, known as the Father of Medicine, developed a diagnostic technique that used color, and in Christ's time, medical practitioners believed that different-colored plasters placed over wounds would help the healing process. The Chinese used and continue to use color for diagnostic purposes and look at the color of various parts of the body to determine conditions of health. In the 20th century, credit has been given to Edward D. Babbitt, Rudolph Steiner, and Dr. Rowland Hunt for continuing research and development of color therapy. Today, many color therapy practices have been established all over the world.

Color is a sensation in our consciousness. Objects are actually colorless and we see wavelengths of light reflected by the object. Some wavelengths are absorbed and others are reflected. A yellow object absorbs all wavelengths except yellow, which is reflected in the eye. Not all of us translate color in the same way. Individuals can perceive color differently. So, the experience of color is subjective. The color we see develops in three stages: physical—the energy of the light emits color vibrations; physiological—the eye's photosensitive cells transform the vibrations into nerve impulses received by the optical nerve center, where color is born; psychological—the nerve center gives us color perception and all of its influences.

Color exerts a tremendous amount of psychological and physiological influence on us. Color and light travel through the eye via the retina, to the brain and the hypothalamus. The hypothalamus is believed to control the physiological expressions of our emotions, as well as the pituitary gland, one of the most complex structures of the body. It stimulates and regulates hormonal and neuro-chemical functions. It also controls involuntary functions and influences our moods. Both the hypothalamus and the pituitary gland are susceptible to the influences of color and light, which explains why we are affected by color.

Color is an integral part of our daily life—from the clothes we wear to the environment that surrounds us. In the early 1900s, European studies in a mental hospital showed how colors could calm hyperactivity and reduce depression.[2] Recent prison studies have shown that inmates are less aggressive when they are in rooms of a particular color, such as light pink and they could be made more aggressive with the use of other colors, such as red.[3] Black, a color associated with death and tragedy, was the color of the Blackfriars Bridge in London, known for its high rate of suicides. When it was painted green, the suicides decreased by one-third.[4]

Color Influences Us

There are seven colors in the visible light spectrum or, as we see it, the rainbow. An easy way to remember these colors is by the acronym, ROY G. BIV. It stands for Red, Orange, Yellow, Green, Blue, Indigo, Violet. (White reflects all light and is the presence of all color. Black absorbs all light and is the absence of all color.)

Red

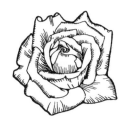 Of all the colors, red is the most powerful. It represents life, enthusiasm, love, celebration, courage, will power, and leadership. Wearing red makes one feel stronger and more dynamic. Red foods are warming and vitalizing. Red should not be used in rooms of the anxious or fearful, as it will aggravate them. Red can be used to periodically boost the energy level but should not be used continually unless the room is for physical activity such as exercising. Red stimulates the appetite, has aphrodisiac qualities, increases the blood pressure, and induces thirst. It stimulates and tones the nervous system. People

who benefit most from red are the anemic and the subdued with lack of vitality. The color is not good for people who are feverish or have an excitable temperament. Red excites the psyche. It inspires and helps create new ideas and can help in overcoming feelings of depression, fear, and inertia.

Orange

Orange represents enthusiasm, health, and happiness. Tints and shades of orange are excellent in rooms for socializing, therapeutic work, and food service. It is a good mixture of the vitalizing red and the intellectual yellow. Orange foods are often high in vitamin A. Orange promotes rejuvenation at a cellular-building level. It can raise the blood pressure, increase the heart rate, and warm the hands and feet. Orange promotes optimism and relieves depression. It is excellent for relieving negative emotional states.

Yellow

Yellow represents the intellect, knowledge, mental clarity, curiosity, cheerfulness, and happiness. It is awakening and inspiring. Yellow has often been the color of ceremonial clothing. Wearing yellow provides protection especially against viruses and infection. Yellow is highly visible and "brighter" than white. It will lighten up dimly lit rooms. Use yellow in rooms where mental clarity is desired. Yellow strengthens nerves and stimulates the appetite and mental activity. It promotes vitamin A absorption. It is excellent for people who are too serious or who take things too hard. It promotes balance and lightens the spirit. Yellow stimulates separateness so it is not good for people who are lonely.

Green

Green represents healing, harmony, prosperity, security, stability, and nature. It is detoxifying and cleansing. Wearing green makes you feel stable and secure. Green foods are generally thought to be detoxifiers and cleansers. Green rooms promote the feeling of cleanliness. The color is excellent used in rooms where cooperation is desired. Green is pacifying, and people tend to slow down in its presence. It reduces nervousness, muscle tension, eye strain, and pain. It builds the physical body and relaxes the nervous system. Green can relieve and heal emotions such as grief, fear, or jealousy.

Blue

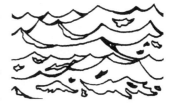

Blue is the color of introspection and encourages introvertedness. It is the coldest color and most people's favorite color. Wearing blue represents conformity. Very often blue is the color of uniforms. For rooms, blue is restful and sedating and makes them seem larger. Blue increases metabolism and promotes growth; calms the mind and sedates the emotions; relieves inflammations and slows the action of the heart. Blue helps prevent sleeplessness. It is a pain killer, heals and cools burns, and relieves itching. It can relieve high blood pressure. It is excellent for concentration. The color blue is not recommended for overly serious people or those experiencing acute depression.

Indigo

Indigo, the darkest color of the spectrum, is very similar to the characteristics of blue in both physical and psychological effects with some influences from violet, such as inspiration. Indigo promotes devotion, clear and logical thought, and present awareness.

Violet

Violet represents independence, royalty, spiritual vitality, and personal power. It is a creative color. Violet rooms are feminine and poetic. They are not good for depressed people. Violet is cooling, astringent, and relaxing to the physical body. It is good for the eyes. It helps overcome sluggish conditions and is a restorative for the nerves. Violet decreases pain sensitivity, lowers blood pressure, and dilates veins. Violet builds creativity and promotes spirituality.

Color and Food

Red   Red foods are stimulating. They are not recommended for people with high blood pressure.

Yellow   Yellow foods are laxative.

Green   Green plant foods are for rejuvenating and rebuilding.

Blue   Blue foods settle the nervous system and are cooling.

Purple   Purple foods are calming and have the added benefit of being inspiring.

Colors and Themes

- Clear colors are the most uplifting.
- Dark colors are serious or depressing.
- Warm colors are productive and energetic.
- Cool colors are soothing and relaxing.

Color and Mental States

Red   Passion, motivation, persistence, gratitude, resentment, hate, irritation, anger

Orange   Outgoing and assertive nature (sometimes overbearing), enthusiasm, creativity, joy

Yellow   Hope, intelligence, cheerfulness, open-mindedness, wisdom, decisiveness, deception, vindictiveness

Green   Sharing, generosity, cooperation, understanding, security, harmony, indifference, over-cautiousness, jealousy, prejudice

Blue   Aspiration, devotion, trust, serenity, doubt, complacency, melancholy

Purple   Dignity, self-respect, oneness, pride, arrogance, forgetfulness

ℋ
For Skin Care

Color can be used during your daily routine of cleansing and toning to benefit both the skin and the psyche. You will need a small light fixture, in front of which are placed different colored transparent gels (thin, translucent sheets of color). These are available from art supply stores. Use the different colored rays of light only for the time it would normally take you to complete the following steps, not longer. Direct the light ray to the ceiling.

Step 1   Use the color lavender in the room as you apply facial compresses as a pre-cleanse treatment. This aids in the relaxation process.

Step 2   During the cleansing process, use the color green.

Step 3   During the toning process:
Use the color red or orange if you have underactive skin;
Use the color yellow if you have normal skin;
Use the color green if you have oily skin;
Use the color blue if you have blemished or sensitive skin.

Color can also be used in skin care to enhance the beneficial effects of water applications. Wrap a transparent color gel (color of your choice) around a glass jar of water and place it in the sun for four hours. This creates water with the vibrational quality of the specific color you chose. This water can be used in a compress, as a toner, or in a facial mister. Red stimulates circulation, maintains the color of the skin, and gives energy to the tissues. Do not use red on inflamed conditions. Orange relieves congestion, stimulates circulation, and maintains the luster of the skin. Green is balancing and freshens the skin. Blue is calming and cooling and very good for acne or irritated skin. According to Ayurveda, blue can also be used to help relieve hyperpigmentation of the skin.

NOTE: Ruth Strock from the Color Research Institute in San Francisco states that stimulating colors should not be used by anyone with heart problems, and violet or blue should not be used by anyone who is depressed.[5]

Recommended Reading

Color Your Life, Howard and Dorothy Sun (New York: Ballantine Books, 1992).

The Reflexology and Color Therapy Workbook, Pauline Wills (Great Britain: Element Books Limited, 1992).

The Healing Power of Color, Betty Wood (Rochester, VT: Destiny Books, 1992).

12

Exercise

Whenever possible, go outdoors in simple clothing. When the weather permits, walk barefoot on grass, beach, or soil. Go on regular outings, especially to beautiful natural areas. A half-hour walk each day activates circulation and energy flow and helps keep the hair and skin fresh and beautiful.
　　　　　—Aveline Kushi, Diet for Natural Beauty

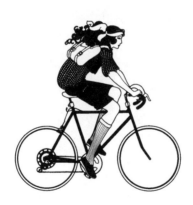

For Health & Well-Being

The human body is designed for action and movement. It wears faster from disuse than it does from use, and operates better with more work than less. Health experts, physicians, and our own bodies tell us that we need to exercise if we want to be physically fit and healthy. In fact, exercise is probably the best way to improve physical and mental energy as well as emotional well-being. This is no wonder when we review the tremendous benefits that result from regular physical activity and movement. Remember, no matter how well you eat or manage stress, what you weigh, or how you live, you are not healthy if you are not reasonably physically fit.

The Benefits of Exercise

❧ Exercise is good for the heart. It strengthens the heart muscle and increases the rate and quality of circulation. Exercise decreases the risk of heart disease; in fact, it is the number one preventive measure. Exercise protects the heart against stressful situations because it makes the heart more resilient. Exercise also lowers the heart rate, which means the heart muscle works more efficiently, beating slower per minute and returning to its resting rate sooner after exercise. Exercise lowers blood pressure, and increases the elasticity of the blood vessels, making them less likely to rupture.

❧ Exercise is good for the bones. It makes them less brittle, with less demineralization. People who are very inactive (such as the bed-ridden) suffer from demineralization, but people who are aerobically active do not experience this type of bone problem. (The impact of feet contacting the ground promotes the absorption of minerals in the bones.)

❧ Exercise improves mental health by promoting clearer thinking, confidence, and creativity. It is common for people to experience more tranquility, better concentration, and increased memory capabilities. This improved mental state is believed to occur for two reasons: a) There is an increase of oxygen to the brain, and b) The body produces endorphins, which reduce pain and can heighten mental awareness. People often feel exhilarated when they exercise and can experience a "second wind" without physical discomfort during an extended exercise period such as marathon running. After a hard work-out, most people feel relaxed, refreshed, and energized.

꙰ Exercise improves lung function. More blood is oxygenated and there is increased air flow through the nasal passages.

꙰ Exercise improves the strength and efficiency of the internal organs due to the increased circulation and internal massage created by physical movement.

꙰ Exercise improves elimination by stimulating body processes. The sooner wastes and toxins are eliminated from the body, the better. The intestinal tract is stimulated, helping to prevent solid wastes from staying in the intestines too long and preventing toxins from re-absorbing into the body. Exercise helps the skin and the lungs, which are also eliminative organs, to throw off more wastes and to do it more efficiently. The better the elimination—the cleaner the body.

꙰ Exercise makes the body more resilient and resistant to the adverse effects of unhealthy living habits such as poor diet or too much alcohol consumption.

꙰ Exercise relieves and often eliminates minor depression. It is said that exercise does not *cure* depression; rather, it is the lack of exercise that causes depression.

꙰ Exercise can relax, strengthen, and stretch muscles to handle more physical and mental demands of life.

꙰ Exercise promotes weight loss in three ways. 1) Calories, which are units to measure the energy value of food, must be used by the body when they are consumed or they will be stored as fat. Exercise helps to use up extra calories (those not used for body functions) before they are stored as fat. 2) Exercise promotes weight loss because it can suppress or normalize the appetite, helping to prevent overeating and bingeing. 3) Exercise increases the rate of metabolism so that *more* calories are used and less stored as fat.

The effect of this increased rate lasts beyond the exercise period, so you can reap the rewards for hours, even on the next day.

❦ For Skin Care

Though all of the benefits listed above positively affect the complexion, there are benefits from exercising that are more specific to the skin. If you exercise regularly:

❦ The skin is firmer and better nourished due to the increased circulation that brings more oxygen and nutrients to the skin.

❦ The aging process is delayed. All the characteristics of aging such as wrinkles, sallowness, and poor circulation are improved with exercise.

❦ Exercise calms the nerves and relieves stress that can deplete the complexion. It increases your resistance to stress and relieves pent-up tensions and minor worries.

❦ A good night's sleep is important for the vitality of the skin. Exercise promotes better sleep, increasing the ability to fall asleep and allowing for a deeper, more revitalizing sleep.

Getting Going

Though most health-conscious people would like to exercise on a regular basis, many complain that it is not easy to find the time, get started, and then stay committed. *Before you begin any work-out or physical activity program, you should get your doctor's approval.* After that, the suggestions below can help you stay on your exercise program.

❦ Exercise with a friend. You can provide support for each other and it is much more fun to have the companionship.

❦ Schedule your exercise time into your weekly itinerary by writing it on your calendar, just as you would any other appointment. A good time for a work-out is after work to release tensions and before dinner because it suppresses your appetite. The afternoon is the best time for stretching-type exercises, when the body is more limber.

❋ Keep your exercise goal simple so that it is attainable and you can be successful. If you set your goal too high, you may feel over-whelmed or over-committed.

❋ Your choice of activity should fit your personality and be something that you enjoy. Some suggestions are jogging, jumping rope, walking, hiking, swimming, rowing, folk-dancing, aerobics, and biking.

❋ Vary your choice of exercise so that you promote *flexibility* (such as stretching or yoga); *strength* (such as weight training or resistance exercises); and *endurance* for cardiovascular fitness (such as walking, dancing, cycling, or jogging).

❋ Be certain that your exercise program does not bore you. It should not make you feel uncomfortable or take up more time than you are willing to commit—these factors can easily defeat your efforts.

❋ Set up a reward system. For example, if you stick to your exercise plan for a month, you have earned a new dress.

❋ Periodically re-read The Benefits of Exercise listed at the beginning of this chapter to remind yourself how important exercise really is!

❋ And, if that isn't enough—here's a reminder of the physical and psychological problems that *can be avoided* with regular exercise.

    a. Bone deterioration
    b. Internal organs not functioning at their optimum
    c. Unfit heart muscle
    d. Weak body muscles
    e. Devitalized skin
    f. Rise in blood pressure
    g. Deterioration of mental health & minor depression
    h. Chronic fatigue
    i. Premature aging

j.   Inadequate flexibility leading to physical injuries
k.   Low back pain
l.   Build-up of tension and stress
m. Tendency to be overweight

Recommended Reading

Stretching, Bob Anderson (Bolinas, CA: Shelter Publications, 1980).

The 12-Minute Total Body Workout, Joyce L. Vedral, Ph.D. (New York: Warner Books, 1989).

Lilias, Yoga & Your Life, Lilias Folan (New York: MacMillan Publishing, 1981).

13

Herbal Therapy

We in the west are starting to regain the recognition of connection with nature, of the profound links between all aspects of life. The use of herbs in healing is but one aspect of the oneness in life that is planet Earth.
—David Hoffman, The Herbal Handbook

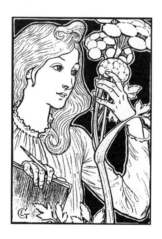

For Health & Well-Being

Using herbs to heal and tend the body is one of the oldest forms of medicine practiced by humankind. Herbs have been used throughout history—at least 5,000 years ago in ancient Egypt, China, and India; in the days of Hippocrates before Christ; in Rome during the first century; and by the Catholic Church in the second century. In the Bible, it is stated in Ezekiel 47:12, "...and the fruit thereof shall be for meat, and the leaf thereof for medicine." Many of the most important drugs used today were derived from herbs such as aspirin from white willow bark, opiate narcotics from the opium poppy, digitalis from foxgloves, and quinine from the bark of the cinchona tree.

In the late 1500s, an era began in England known as the Great Age of Herbals. Large volumes were written about the medical properties of herbs. Herbal usage continued for many years and was then brought to the New World. Thomas Jefferson grew a variety of herbs at Monticello. During the mid-20th century, in the industrialized cultures, the use of herbal medicine declined significantly, being replaced by chemical pharmaceuticals made in laboratories. By the latter part of the 20th century, herbal medicine experienced a "comeback," being favored by lay people seeking a more "natural" lifestyle and being recognized by the medical establishment as effective in certain applications. In less industrialized countries, the use of herbal therapy has remained constant. In fact, seventy-five percent of the people in the world employ healing herbs as their primary source of medicine.[1]

An herb is a plant or part of a plant that is used for its medicinal, culinary, or aromatic qualities. Every part of a plant can be used—the leaf, root, bark, flower, stalk, fruit, and seed. The time of harvesting, the soil, the water availability, the time of day, and the season will all have a bearing on the quality of a plant's medicinal characteristics. Herbs can be used in a variety of ways such as infused as a tea, extracted as a tincture, pressed into a tablet, mixed with water for a poultice, or melted with beeswax for a salve. Herbs can be taken internally or applied externally.

The most common therapeutic uses for herbs are:

❧ To cleanse and purify the body.

❧ To normalize body function by helping to regulate and tone the glands and organs.

❧ To provide nutrients in the form of vitamins, minerals, and trace minerals.

❧ To maintain good health and to raise the energy level of the body.

❧ To support the body's immune system by stimulating natural defense systems.

How to Obtain Herbs

1. Collect them yourself. Collecting herbs requires the ability to identify the plants and harvest them during the optimum season and time of day. This can be an enjoyable hobby but may not be practical for most people. In addition, the herbs you want to use may not grow in your area.

2. Grow them yourself. Starting an herb garden in your yard can supply you with fresh, fragrant herbs for your medicinal, culinary, and cosmetic needs. It is a delightful way to use them and great for people who like to garden and have the space and time.

3. Buy them. This is the quickest and most practical way to begin working with herbs, but it is the most expensive. You also must rely on the supplier and trust that the herbs are fresh and that they have been properly harvested, prepared, and stored. If you purchase your herbs, as most people do, find a reputable supplier. Herbs are available at most natural food stores and by mail order.

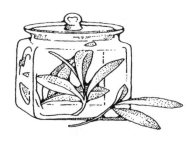

Drying & Storing Herbs

If you choose to collect or grow herbs yourself and keep them for future use, they need to be properly dried and stored. They should be dried as quickly as possible after harvesting to preserve the plant and its potency. Herbs are best dried in a temperature that is cool to warm. The location should be dark and dry with circulating air. Herbs dry well when laid on paper and turned regularly; hung upside down; or put on racks. Home dehydrators work very well for this purpose. Be sure the herbs are completely dry before storing them or else they will become moldy.

The therapeutic qualities of herbs are destroyed by light, heat, and air. To prevent this, store your dried herbs in an air-tight container, out of direct sunlight, and in a cool area. Label them with their name, date of storage, and intended use. Replace them when necessary. Be aware that even when herbs are properly dried and stored, they are not effective indefinitely. Leaves and flowers last about a year. Roots, barks, and stems will last up to three years.

Solvents Used for Herbal Preparations

Solvents are used to extract the chemical constituents and therapeutic qualities from an herb and make them available in a liquid solution. The most common solvents are water, alcohol, vinegar, oil, and glycerin. Each has its advantages and disadvantages. When working with herbs and solvents use ceramic, glass, or stainless steel containers. Do not use aluminum or plastics because they interfere with the essence of herbs.

Water

Water is the most often used solvent. From the plant, water will extract vitamins, minerals, starches, and gums as well as sugars, acids, tannins, and some volatile oils. Water does not preserve the herb, so a water-solvent preparation must be refrigerated and made fresh every few days. Water preparations of herbs can be done with an infusion, a warm water infusion, a solar infusion, or a decoction.

An *infusion* is used for lighter, less dense plants such as flowers and leaves. The standard measurement for an infusion is one cup of water to one rounded teaspoon of dried herb. To make an infusion: pour boiling water over the herb and cover the container. Steep for a minimum of five minutes and a maximum of forty-five minutes, depending on the desired use and qualities to be extracted. The longer the herb is steeped, the more constituents are extracted. A strong infusion uses one cup of water to one rounded tablespoon of dried herb. When you prepare a cup of tea, you are making an herbal infusion. (It is not advisable to use tap water when working with herbs. There are many elements found in tap water today such as chlorine that are undesirable for therapeutic preparations. Instead, use spring water or distilled water.) A *warm water infusion* is used to retain vitamin C or other highly volatile essences that are inherent in a particular plant. To make a warm water infusion: pour one cup of warm water over one teaspoon of herb. Cover and allow to steep several hours or overnight. A *solar infusion* can be used for leaves and flowers, and is excellent for fresh herbs. To make a solar infusion: put one-fourth cup of herb in three cups of water in a quart (or larger) glass container. Close with a tight-fitting lid. Place in a warm, sunny spot for several hours and then strain and bottle for use. *A decoction* is used for harder plant material such as roots, barks, and stems to extract minerals, gums, resins, and saline substances. To make a decoction: place one teaspoon of herb in a pan with one cup of water. Bring to a boil and simmer for fifteen minutes (minimum) to forty-five minutes (maximum).

Alcohol

Alcohol is the second most commonly used solvent. It extracts resins, tannins, organic acids, alkaloids, balsams, and glucocides. Alcohol is especially useful as a solvent because it preserves the extraction. Commonly used alcohols are brandy, rum, and vodka. The higher the alcohol content, the greater the extracting capabilities. One hundred proof vodka works very well and is good for internal and external purposes. Herbal preparations made with alcohol are called tinctures, and they are practical because they have a long shelf life (thirty to forty years), are easy to use, easy to make, and require little storage space (as opposed to bulk herbs). To make a tincture: put one or two ounces of dried herb in one pint of rum, brandy or vodka. Use a wide-mouthed glass jar with a tight-fitting lid. Place the jar in a warm spot in the house (not sunny) for fourteen days. Shake it gently every day and then strain and bottle. Label your tinctures with the storage date, herb name, and intended use. In formulas, tinctures are generally used just a few drops at a time because they are concentrated. However, because each batch can vary in strength, you will need to experiment with the dosage. One-fourth to one teaspoon of tincture will equal the strength of one cup of tea.

Vinegar

Vinegar is also used for tinctures. Apple cider vinegar is best but white vinegar may also be used. Vinegar has preserving qualities but it is not as strong as alcohol, so a vinegar tincture will last up to one year. Though not as powerful a solvent as alcohol, vinegar imparts its own qualities to the preparation. Apple cider vinegar has vitamins, minerals, and certain enzymes. When used externally, It replaces and supports the natural acidic nature of the skin. A vinegar tincture is made in the same way as the alcohol tinctures.

Oil

Oil is sometimes used as a solvent for herbal extractions but it is not powerful and the herb will leave only its subtle presence in the oil. Any oil can be used to infuse herbs. Oils that are especially good for cosmetics are olive, almond, and apricot which can be used separately or blended together. To make an oil infusion: place three ounces of dried herbs in a quart jar and fill the jar with oil. Cover tightly and place the jar in a warm, sunny spot. Shake daily for one to two weeks. If you are having very hot days (85 degrees or more), the oil should be done in five days. Strain, bottle, label properly, and then refrigerate. An herbal oil can also be made by placing three ounces of herb in the top of a double boiler. Cover with one quart of oil. Simmer for twenty to forty-five minutes. Keep checking the oil for a rich fragrance, which will indicate it is finished. Strain, bottle, label, and refrigerate.

Glycerin

Glycerin is a constituent of all oils and fats, both animal and vegetable. It is a good preservative but does not have the versatility and effectiveness of alcohol. Glycerin is, however, more soothing, nurturing, and nourishing. It extracts fixed alkalies, minerals, vitamins, and gums as well as starches, acids, oils, and tannins. To use glycerin as a solvent: dissolve one part glycerin in three parts water. Soak two to four ounces of dried, ground herb in one pint of the water/glycerin mixture. Place in a warm spot for fourteen days, shaking daily. Strain, bottle, label, and store.

For Skin Care

Herbs are used in skin care to soothe, relax, and soften the complexion. They also nourish and cleanse. Specific herbs can stimulate and rejuvenate the complexion. Herbs used in skin care products are usually in the form of extracts or infusions added to moisturizers, cleansers, toners, facial misters, or masks.

The most popular cosmetic herbs are arnica, calendula, chamomile, comfrey, elderflower, ginkgo biloba, ginseng, green tea, horsetail, lavender, nettle, peppermint, rose, rosemary, St. Johnswort, witch hazel, and yarrow. Listed below are the uses of these herbs in skin care products. (More about each of these herbs can be found in Chapter 6, "Super Natural Ingredients for Skin Care.")

To sooth   Chamomile, lavender, arnica, calendula, elderflower, witch hazel, rose, green tea

To relax   Chamomile, lavender, St. Johnswort

To soften   Chamomile, lavender, St. Johnswort, rose

To nourish	Ginkgo biloba, comfrey, ginseng, horsetail, St. Johnswort
To cleanse	Chamomile, lavender, nettle, rosemary, arnica, calendula, comfrey, elderflower, peppermint, yarrow
To stimulate	Rosemary, peppermint, nettle, ginkgo biloba
To rejuvenate	Arnica, calendula, chamomile, comfrey, ginkgo biloba, ginseng, lavender, rosemary, green tea

Recommended Reading

The Herb Book, John Lust (New York: Bantam Books, 1974).

Herbal Medicine, Dian Dincin Buchman (New York: David McKay Company, Inc.,1979).

The Herbal Handbook, David Hoffman (Rochester, VT: Healing Arts Press, 1987).

14

Hydrotherapy

=====

*Water is the most healing of all remedies
and the best of all cosmetics.*

—*Arab proverb*

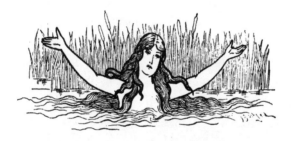

For Health & Well-Being

H ydrotherapy, literally "water remedy," has been used for thousands of years and is considered *the* oldest natural form of medicine. Water was used for massaging and cleansing the sick at the temples of Asclepius, the Greek god of medicine. Hippocrates used water to reduce fevers and treated a variety of illnesses with baths of different temperatures. Modern-day hydrotherapists use water in its varied forms (ice, liquid, steam—all of them having their specific function in healing and maintaining health) to energize, relax, and promote stamina as well as tone and detoxify the body.

Hydrotherapy has remained popular for centuries primarily because it is accessible, convenient, and so effective. This may be due to water's ability to increase the body's natural defense mechanisms. Cold water is restorative, re-energizing, and helps build resistance to disease. Hot water is soothing, relaxing, and sedating. In *The Complete Book of Water Therapy* Dian Dincin Buchman states, "What is exceptional about water therapy [hydrotherapy] is that it works with each person's own nature. Water therapy acts in a positive way, and never destroys valuable internal flora, nor does it deplete the energy of internal organs. Water therapy *creates* circulation and overcomes sluggishness; it also unblocks an energy barrier so that the body can function in a freer and more normal fashion."[1] Its treatment is painless and has no damaging side effects.

For Skin Care

Hydrotherapy is extraordinarily effective when used in a personal skin care program for improving the complexion. There are three valuable and enjoyable ways of using water externally: compressing, steaming, and misting. These can be part of your daily routine and will result in beautifully clean, hydrated, and conditioned skin. Water, the universal "elixir of life" is one of our most valuable beauty aids.

Compresses

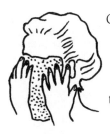

Compresses—folded cloths immersed in water and then applied to the skin—are a good way the gain some of the benefits of water. See Chapter 3 for details about using compresses in your skin care program to cleanse, hydrate, and condition your skin. Extreme temperatures, either very hot or very cold water, are not recommended on the skin, especially the face.

Water Temperatures

Cool water tightens, slows down the glandular activity, decreases circulation and calms inflammation. Warm water relaxes the tissues, encourages glandular activity, and increases circulation.

Normal skin Use cool or warm compresses.
Oily skin Use cool to tepid compresses.
Dry skin Use warm compresses.
Combination skin Use warm compresses.
Sensitive skin Use tepid or warm compresses.
Blemished skin Use cool to tepid compresses.
Mature skin Use warm compresses.

Herbal infusions can be added to the basin water for compresses to nourish and condition the skin as well as help alleviate skin problems. Choose a blend appropriate for your skin type. (See Chapter 7, "Making Your Own Skin Care Products.") After you have thoroughly mixed the dried herbs, make a strong tea using two tablespoons of herbs to one cup of boiling water. Cover and allow to steep for thirty minutes. Strain, then pour the tea into the basin and add warm or cool water, whichever is appropriate for your skin type, and apply the compress as usual.

Essential oils can be used with facial compresses to create a wonderful treatment that provides the benefits of both hydrotherapy and aromatherapy. See Chapter 9 for more on aromatherapy.

Steam

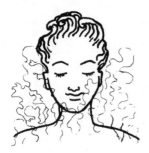

Steam is the gaseous state of water that results from heating it to a high temperature. Facial steaming is appropriate for most types of skin and can be used on a regular basis to garner some of the benefits of hydrotherapy. You will need to purchase a small facial steamer at a department or drug store. (The face-over-the-pot-method is not recommended.) Steaming time and frequency depends on the skin type. See Chapter 3 (under "Special Treatments") for details about facial steaming.

Misting

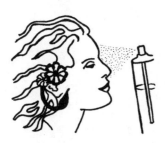

Facial misting is used to refresh and hydrate the skin. Used regularly, in conjunction with a moisturizer that contains a good humectant, it can soften and even eliminate superficial lines on the face, particularly around the eyes. It is especially important to mist the face in dry climates, air-conditioned rooms, and airplanes, where there is little moisture in the air. Loss of moisture in the facial skin is a cause of premature wrinkling, and the misting form of hydrotherapy can help counteract this.

Misters may contain rosewater, aloe vera, floral waters, or herbal extracts. These special ingredients, combined with water, make an effective hydrating and conditioning treatment for the skin. However, water is the most important ingredient here and is a genuine moisturizer. (See Chapter 7, "Making Your Own Skin Care Products.")

When the weather is warm, misting need not be limited to the face. Misting the arms, legs, and shoulders can prevent you from feeling "wilted" in the heat. If you spend time in the sun (with a sunscreen, of course), misting will keep your skin cool and hydrated.

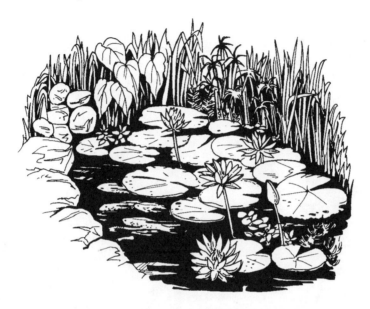

Recommended Reading

The Complete Book of Water Therapy, Dian Dincin Buchman (New York: E.P Dutton, 1979).

Modern Magic of Natural Healing with Water Therapy, J.V. Cerney (New York: Parker Publishing Company, Inc., 1975).

15

Massage

Increased circulation is one of the key ingredients in the massage recipe. It steps up the flow of blood and oxygen to the entire body, leaving a person feeling relaxed, stress-free, and revitalized.
> —Alana Schneider, Journalist

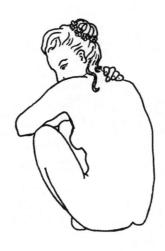

✿

For Health & Well Being

M assage is the use of the hands to manipulate the skin and muscles of the body. The word "massage" is derived from roots meaning "to knead" or "to handle." Massage (and touching) can be used as a supportive and therapeutic technique for the physical body as well as the psyche. The chemicals produced in the brain when a person is massaged can also change moods or feelings. It can soothe, relax, and relieve pain. The technique of using the hands therapeutically on the skin of oneself or another is universal and perhaps even instinctual. If we bruise or hurt ourselves, an immediate reaction is to put our hands there. If a friend or a loved one is hurt, we will reach out with our hands to hold the area or perhaps offer a hug.

Massage and "healing touch" have been used by cultures all over the world throughout history. The earliest records are from China, when massage was used as "a welcome relief for exhausted heros."[1] Hippocrates used massage as one of his methods of healing. A Swede by the name of Per Henrik Ling studied and taught massage and popularized it in Europe in the early 1800s. Massage as used today in its variety of forms has evolved from techniques learned from the East and techniques developed in the West. A diversity of movements or strokes range from light, gentle touch to a heavier, more manipulative one. Long, gliding strokes as well as kneading, circular, and tapping motions are commonly used. Though there are many schools of thought and methods of massage, they all are based on the fundamental healing aspects of hands touching the skin.

✿

For Skin Care

NOTE: Because this part of the book is written for self-care, the following information in limited to those techniques that do not require a second person.

Massage is used today in professional skin care (face and body) because of its remarkable ability to increase circulation and reduce stress. Following is a list of the important benefits of massage as they relate to the nurturing of the skin, the complexion, and the psyche.

- Massage dilates the blood vessels, thereby improving circulation.

- Muscles are relaxed and tension is relieved by massage.

- Massage increases the blood supply to muscles without adding to their load of toxic lactic acid (which is produced through voluntary muscle contractions).

- Massage may have a sedative, stimulating, or exhausting effect on the nervous system, depending on the type and length of massage.

- By improving general circulation, massage increases nutrition to the tissues. It is accompanied or followed by an increased interchange of substances between blood and tissue cells, which can heighten tissue metabolism.

- Fat cells in the subcutaneous tissues can be reduced in size by massage.

- Massage helps the skin to become soft and pliable.

- The skin's glandular activities are stimulated by massage.

- Massage stimulates and strengthens the muscle fibers.

- Massage helps the body cope with the stresses of the environment by relieving tension.

- Massage helps to remove waste products from the body.

- Because circulation is increased, massage can bring better color to the face, along with more oxygen and nutrients.

- Hemoglobin levels increase, which means there is more oxygen reaching more places in the body.

- Massage makes you feel good.

Using Massage for Skin Care at Home

NOTE: Massage should not be used for skin care if there are skin eruptions, rashes or bruises.

1. A good, stimulating head massage increases circulation to the head as well as the facial skin. Heavy *facial* massage is not recommended because it can pull and drag the skin, encouraging wrinkles and sagging. Acupressure is the preferred method of direct facial stimulation. See Chapter 8, "Acupressure" for more details.

2. A thorough ear massage stimulates circulation to the head area and stimulates reflex points in the ears that benefit the entire body.

3. Massage one hand with the other and then reverse. This feels wonderful and also stimulates the reflex points that benefit and correlate to the entire body.

4. Massage the feet well, concentrating on the areas that are particularly good for the skin such as the lung and the intestinal area. (See Chapter 18, "Reflexology.")

5. Drop the head to the chest and massage the neck and the shoulders. This is an area that commonly holds tension and a deep massage can bring relief and relaxation.

6. Lubricate the skin around the eyes with a moisturizer or facial oil. Massage gently, going around the eyes in a circle, following the muscle and using the underlying bone as support. This is the only sliding massage technique recommended for use directly on the face, used to increase circulation and prevent wrinkles. It is described in detail in Chapter 8, "Acupressure." It is used to increase circulation and prevent wrinkles.

Recommended Reading

The Massage Book, George Downing (New York: Random House, 1972).
The Complete Book of Massage, Clare Maxell-Hudson (New York: Random House, 1988).
The Book of Massage, Lucinda Lidell (New York: Simon and Schuster, 1984).

16

Nutrition

A rapidly growing number of people are regaining their health through simple, natural eating. They have decided to take charge of their own health and life.
—*Annemarie Colbin,* Food and Healing

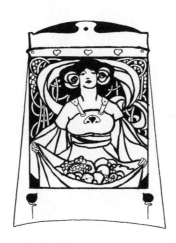

For Health & Well-Being

Nutrition is used therapeutically today by lay people as well as health care professionals to help solve physical and psychological problems and to maintain and support good health. Specific diets are used successfully for certain health conditions such as diabetes, high blood pressure, heart irregularities, arthritis, and obesity. Breakthroughs in nutritional therapy have also helped people with depression and anxiety.

The food we eat replenishes the body with vital energy. Dr. James Braly, a medical doctor that specializes in nutrition and immunology, stated, "What we put in our mouths is the fuel for our bodies; it is the most crucial determinant of our level of performance, of how well and how long we will live."[1]

There are many schools of thought today on the best way to nourish ourselves. Knowing which approach is best for you will take some exploring, but it is so important to eat well that it should be given conscious attention and top priority. Your chosen dietary philosophy should be appropriate for your current physical and mental condition as well as your taste and preference. It should make you feel comfortable and satisfied. If you have health problems, seeking the advice of a health professional is recommended because changing your diet could help restore your health. If you have no existing health problems but want to take a more active role in your well-being, educate yourself, investigate, and choose a guided practice of eating. You will have many options from which to choose such as vegetarian (vegan or strict vegetarian), lacto-vegetarian, ovo-lacto-vegetarian, fruitarian, allergy-elimination, whole food diet, macrobiotic, mucousless, or Basic 4 food group.

There is no such thing as "an average person" when it comes to nutritional needs, so guidelines suggested by the RDAs (recommended daily allowances) may be inadequate for *your* nutritional needs. In addition, your nutritional needs will change over the course of your life. Your optimal diet is determined by current physical and mental conditions, food allergies, and preferences. The factors listed below may influence your present nutritional needs.

1. Genetic predisposition (ancestry, heredity)

2. Environment

3. Age

4. Body size and type

5. Stress levels

6. Physical activity levels

7. Allergies

8. Illnesses

9. Medications

10. Sleep pattern

11. Resistance to disease

12. Ability of digestive tract to absorb and use nutrients

13. Pregnancy

14. Cigarette smoking

15. Alcohol consumption

In addition to good, wholesome food that nurtures and supports your mental and physical health, supplementation may be warranted periodically. Many health practitioners feel that taking supplements such as vitamins or minerals in conjunction with good food (not as a substitute) is appropriate today for the following reasons.

1. The current polluted condition of our environment (soil, water, air) puts additional stress on our bodies.

2. The soil is depleted and does not grow plants that are as nutrient-rich as they should be.

3. Many fruits and vegetables are picked for market before they are ripe and fully nutritionally developed.

4. Today's eating habits make it almost impossible to get all the nutrients necessary to maintain optimum health.

5. Food processing such as heating and boiling causes loss of nutrients.

6. Almost everyone today is dealing with mental and physical stress (even exercise) which increases our nutritional needs.

7. Certain medications, such as aspirin, can increase our nutritional needs.

Stress can deplete nutrients, affect our eating habits, and influence the complexion. See Chapter 19, "Managing Stress," under "Nutrition and Supplements," for more about this issue.

Guidelines for Healthy Eating

1. Choose foods that are as close as possible to their natural state—fresh and unprocessed. Avoid food additives such as artificial coloring and flavorings, preservatives, and other processing chemicals. Eat as few dried, canned, frozen, or prepared foods as possible.

2. Choose foods that are in season.

3. Vary your diet. It is important to avoid eating the same things for breakfast, lunch, or dinner every day. If you fall into this habit, you may not get all the nutrients you need and you also increase your chances for developing food allergies.

4. Avoid highly refined foods that are void of nutritional value such as white flour and white sugar products.

5. Your diet may need to change from time to time. Choose a philosophy of eating that works for you and makes you feel good physically and emotionally. Then set realistic goals for yourself to stay on your chosen diet but be aware that you need to periodically change your diet to meet immediate needs. It is important to learn what works well for *you*. It may not be what is currently the most popular.

6. Take your time in making any drastic dietary transitions. If your goal requires that you make ten major changes in your diet, start with one or two at a time.

7. Try to eat only when you are hungry. Eat foods that you like. Eat slowly and chew your food well so that it digests properly. Do not eat when you are emotionally upset and do not overeat. Eat in a relaxed environment and ENJOY! Eating should be a pleasurable experience.

8. Hidden food allergies are very common and not easily recognized. They do not cause a rash or a stuffy nose, which are reactions commonly associated with allergies. In addition, a hidden food allergy reaction may be delayed—causing a problem twenty-four hours later. These characteristics make it very difficult to identify the offending food. You could be eating a very healthy diet, but if you are allergic to the foods, you will not feel well. Hidden food allergy symptoms can be fatigue, skin problems, headaches, poor digestion, and mood swings. For more information about hidden food allergies, contact ImmunoLab in Florida at 1-800-231-9197 or Immuno Diagnostic Laboratories 707-765-6586.

9. Eat consciously. Think about the food you are eating as genuine nourishment. Really taste it and notice the texture and smell. Pay attention to how the food makes you feel, especially after eating. (If you feel very tired after eating, it may be due to food allergies.)

Nutrients Supplied by Our Food

Carbohydrates

Carbohydrates supply most of the energy for the body and also help in the assimilation of other nutrients. Sugar, starch, and cellulose are the main carbohydrates. Sugar is the most easily digested, starch is slightly more difficult, and cellulose is nearly undigestible. Cellulose does not supply energy, but instead, provides bulk for proper elimination. Through digestion, sugars and starches are broken down and converted into glucose, which is used immediately for energy or converted into glycogen and stored in the liver or in muscle tissue. The remainder is converted into fat and stored throughout the body for later use. *(Some sources: fruits, vegetables, breads, cereals, pastas, whole grains.)*

Protein

Protein provides the materials (amino acids) for building tissue in the body and for the production of hormones and enzymes. If carbohydrates and fats are not present, protein can also be used for energy. Excess protein is converted into fat and stored in body tissues. Of the twenty-two different amino acids that the body needs, it is capable of producing fourteen. The other eight, called the "essential amino acids" must come from food. "Complete proteins" contain all eight of these amino acids. Animal protein is a complete protein. Vegetable protein usually is not complete, though there are exceptions such as soybeans. A deficiency of protein in the body can affect the skin by inhibiting healing, slowing down cellular rejuvenation, and possibly contributing to premature aging. *(Some sources: meat, fish, chicken, eggs, dried beans, dairy products.)*

Fats

Fats are a concentrated form of energy, having nearly twice as much as carbohydrates or protein. Fats help the assimilation of certain vitamins in the body and insulate the body from the environment. Fats are the slowest to be digested. Once digested, they break down into fatty acids, which pass through the intestinal wall and into the bloodstream. *(Some sources: butter, oils.)*

Vitamins

Vitamins are essential to life even though they do not provide energy or build tissue. They are considered catalysts for the proper functioning of bodily processes and regulate biochemical reactions. There are both water-soluble and fat-soluble vitamins. Excess water-soluble vitamins are excreted through the urine when not needed by the body. Fat-soluble vitamins are stored in the body and can be used over a period of time. (*Some sources: vegetables, fruits, meats, nuts, grains.*)

Minerals

Minerals are nutrients that work closely with vitamins as catalysts and are also necessary for proper body functioning. Minerals are stored in the body, but deficiencies can result from non-replenished supplies. Macro-minerals are found in large amounts in the body. They are calcium, chlorine, magnesium, phosphorus, potassium, sodium, and sulfur. Micro-minerals are found in tiny amounts but are still essential for good health. They are aluminum, cadmium, copper, fluorine, and iodine. (*Some sources: vegetables, fruits, herbs, molasses.*)

Water

The human body is ninety percent water, the most plentiful substance in the body. Water is necessary for digestion, cooling, internal cleansing, elimination, and the circulation of nutrients to every cell of the body. (*Some sources: fruits, vegetables, juices.*)

For Skin Care

Nutrition plays a vital role in skin care because the condition of our skin is a reflection of our general health. At any given moment, twenty-five percent of the body's blood supply is contained in the skin. The blood supply circulates completely through the body every minute. Thus, there is constant communication between internal functions and the skin itself, with internal imbalance quickly mirrored in the skin.

Because the blood contains the nutrients necessary for good health and a beautiful complexion, it has been said that problems with the skin are a sure sign of poor nutrition. Good health and a beautiful complexion are determined in part by our diet. After all, our skin is not only produced but also nourished by the raw materials that go into our bodies as food. It stands to reason that the quality of the food we eat will play a role in the quality and appearance of our skin.

Vitamins, Minerals & Essential Fatty Acids: Their Role in Skin Care

The following vitamins, minerals, and essential fatty acids are important and used by the body as a whole. However, they also play a specific, crucial role in the health of the skin such as protecting the skin from sun damage, helping to reverse the effects of aging caused by sun damage, and helping to heal wounds and infections. The benefits listed below are in relationship to the skin and do not include every known function for each substance.

Vitamins

Vitamin A (fat-soluble): Necessary for tissue repair, cell renewal and maintenance; helps to keep skin elastic; helps prevent dryness and wrinkling; has anti-oxidant qualities (see Glossary); helps to prevent infection.
Some sources: carrots, squash, spinach, broccoli

Beta Carotene (both water-and oil- soluble forms): Converts to vitamin A when needed; important anti-oxidant; may function as an internal sunscreen.
Some sources: carrots, squash, apricots

Vitamin B complex (water-soluble): Known for its anti-stress capabilities; includes B1, B2, B3, B5, B6, B12, B15, biotin, choline, folic acid, inositol, and PABA; helps metabolize carbohydrates, fats, and protein for energy and tissue repair; necessary for proper digestion and circulation; helps keep the nervous system healthy, so it is especially important in times of stress; supports immune-system function; necessary for cell regeneration and repair to keep the complexion youthful.
Some sources: whole grains, peanuts, leafy vegetables, nutritional yeast

Vitamin C (water-soluble): Necessary for the production of elastin and collagen; necessary for healing and for the formation of red blood cells; necessary for digestion, proper immune function, and the metabolism of other vitamins and

minerals; a powerful anti-oxidant; necessary for the metabolism of carbohydrates, fats and proteins; promotes skin strength and elasticity in blood vessel walls and cell membranes.
Some sources: citrus fruit, bell and chili peppers, vegetables

Vitamin D (fat-soluble): Necessary for the metabolism of calcium and phosphorus.
Some sources: fish liver oils, egg yolk, certain fish

Vitamin E (fat-soluble): Has anti-oxidant qualities; protects the immune system; helps to maintain all tissues; believed to slow the aging of cells; plays a role in cellular respiration and circulation; may help prevent scar formation.
Some sources: cold-pressed vegetable oils, avocadoes, raw nuts and seeds

Vitamin K (fat-soluble): Essential to overall health and vitality; important factor for blood clotting.
Some sources: kelp, alfalfa, yogurt, egg yolks, green leafy vegetables

Bioflavonoids (water-soluble): Once called vitamin P (for permeability) but because they did not fit the exact description of a vitamin, they were re-named "substance P;" powerful anti-oxidant; enhances efficiency of vitamins A and C; reduces inflammation; reduces allergic reactions; reduces and relieves pain; strengthens capillary walls and prevents capillary damage; helps to maintain collagen integrity.
Some sources: solid parts of citrus fruits, black currants, cherries, rosehips

Minerals

Calcium: Necessary for cellular metabolism; helps to heal wounds; important for nerve health—it can calm the nerves. The average body contains about three pounds of calcium.
Some sources: milk, cheese, beans, lentils, figs, cabbage

Chromium: Necessary for metabolism of carbohydrates and fatty acids; may be essential for circulation in the tiny capillaries near the epidermis.
Some sources: brewer's yeast, whole grains, mushrooms, milk products

Copper: Necessary for the formation of red blood cells; supports skin function; helps protect against oxidation damage; helps to strengthen the skin in con-

junction with the production of collagen and elastin; helps to maintain a healthy color to the skin.
Some sources: whole grains, almonds, raisins, most beans

Fluorine: Protects against infection; helps in the formation of bone and dental tissue.
Some sources: fluorinated water, seafood

Iodine: Necessary for the growth and repair of all tissues; important in production of energy.
Some sources: seafood

Iron: Plays a role in oxygen use and energy production; supports the immune system; necessary for protein metabolism; can prevent pale skin; active in cell renewal and the utilization of oxygen in skin cells.
Some sources: liver, leafy green vegetables, blackstrap molasses, prunes, raisins

Magnesium: Necessary for metabolism of carbohydrates and amino acids; plays a role in fatty acid metabolism; aids in proper nerve function; activator of enzyme systems; helps maintain membrane integrity and vascular tone.
Some sources: fresh green vegetables, nuts, soybeans

Manganese: Helps in metabolism of certain vitamins, carbohydrates, fats and proteins; supports anti-oxidant system.
Some sources: whole grains, egg yolk, bananas, beans, celery

Phosphorus: Necessary for tissue growth and repair; necessary for metabolism of calcium, vitamins, carbohydrates, fats, and proteins; helps prevent fatigue.
Some sources: meat, fish, fowl, eggs, nuts, whole grains

Potassium: Plays a role in amino acid metabolism; helps regulate body water balance and elimination of wastes.
Some sources: leafy green vegetables, citrus fruits, tomatoes, whole grains, bananas

Selenium: Has strong anti-oxidant qualities; protects the skin from free radical damage; protects against ultra-violet-induced cell damage; helps preserve skin elasticity.
Some sources: (depends on content in soil) whole grains, broccoli, onion, eggs

Silicon: Present in high quantities in the skin of young adults, decreasing with age; supports skin flexibility, elasticity, and strength.
Some sources: vegetables, whole grains, seafood

Sodium: Necessary for proper digestion; works with potassium to regulate water balance.
Some sources: celery, cheese, seafood, salt, poultry

Sulfur: Smooths, tones and purifies the skin; aids in collagen production and the formation of new cells.
Some sources: meat, fish, legumes, nuts, eggs

Zinc: Necessary for metabolism of B-complex vitamins; supports immune function and proper healing; necessary for essential fatty acid metabolism; helps to limit free radical damage; essential for normal cell growth and repair; plays a role in many of the body's enzyme systems.
Some sources: whole grains, most seafood, sunflower seeds, onions

Essential Fatty Acids (EFAs)

Essential fatty acids were once referred to as vitamin F. There are several EFAs such as eicosapentaenoic acid, docosahexaenoic acid, gamma linolenic acid, linoleic acid, arachidonic acid, and alpha linolenic acid.

Essential Fatty Acids: Necessary for the proper functioning of all tissues and tissue repair, especially the skin (EFAs play an essential role in maintaining healthy skin by holding skin cells together in a water-tight seal and retaining moisture); anti-inflammatory agents; support the body's immune system; form the basic building blocks from which body fats, membranes, and prostaglandins (hormone-like substances) are made; contribute to the skin's ability to hold moisture; vital to every cell membrane in the body; cannot be manufactured by the body, so they must be supplied by in the diet. Essential fatty acid deficiencies include skin dryness and roughness and a tendency for skin problems such as eczema, itchiness, and acne.
Best sources: unsaturated fats such as vegetable oils and seed oils such as evening primrose oil, flax seed oil, olive oil. Saturated animal fats do not contain enough essential fatty acids.

Recommended Reading

The Doctors' Vitamin and Mineral Encyclopedia, Sheldon Saul Hendler, M.D., Ph.D. (New York: Simon and Shuster, 1990).

Food and Healing, Annemarie Colbin (New York: Ballantine Books, 1986).

Diet for Natural Beauty, Aveline Kushi (New York: Japan Publication, Inc., 1991).

Healing with Whole Foods, Paul Pitchford (Berkeley, CA: North Atlantic Books, 1993).

17

Polarity Therapy

A subtle invisible energy is everywhere and sustains all life. Polarity recognizes this energy and the integral nature of the body and mind. It is energy that restores the spent corporeal resources, balances the strained mind, and ultimately lifts the spirits so that man feels whole again.

—Peter Pick, Polarity Therapist

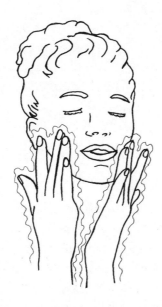

For Health & Well-Being

Polarity Therapy balances the subtle energy of the body. It encourages relaxation, promotes a sense of well-being, and is an excellent way to relieve stress. Developed by Dr. Randolph Stone, Polarity Therapy is the result of years of study and the blending of a variety of natural healing techniques such as acupuncture, herbal medicine, Ayurveda, and yoga. Polarity Therapy is non-manipulative. That is, it does not work on the muscles, bones, or connective tissues. Rather, it works on the subtle energy of the body, removing blocks that prevent the flow of energy. Polarity was designed to help the *whole* person—physically, mentally, and spiritually.

At the core of the Polarity Therapy philosophy is the concept that our bodies are more than just skin, bones, nerves, and parts. This "something more" has been called by other philosophies as the life force, *chi*, soul, and spirit. In Polarity Therapy, it is referred to as "energy."

Involving attitude, body-work, diet, and exercise, Polarity is a complex art that could be the focus of a lifetime of work. Yet Polarity Therapy techniques are effective without a knowledge of the complexities and can be done by anyone. Indeed, many of us use the principles of Polarity Therapy without even knowing it.

For Skin Care

Used in a cosmetic context, Polarity promotes harmony and balance in the body and helps alleviate mental and physical stress. Both of these qualities support a vibrant, healthy complexion. The following simple Polarity exercises are easy, do not take much time, and will leave you feeling revitalized—even after doing just one!

NOTE: The following exercises were taught to the author by a Polarity Therapist, whose name, unfortunately, is not known. She instructed a class at an herbal retreat in mid-1970. The author has used these exercises ever since.

Scissor Kick

With plenty of room around you, lie face down on the floor, with both of your hands under your forehead, palms down. Bend your knees and move them about a foot apart. Your feet are in the air. Swing your feet out and then back again, crossing at the ankles with the right leg in front. Swing out and cross again, with the left leg in front. Do this for 5 minutes, at a slow or quick pace.

This exercise is designed to open and stimulate the energy flow in the body and to build stamina.

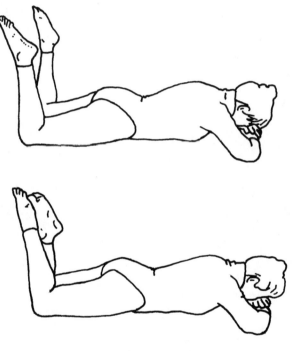

The Basic Squat

Stand erect with your feet about 12 inches apart. Raise up on your toes, raise your arms in front of you at shoulder level (for balance), and then lower yourself to a squatting position. Ideally, your heels should be on the ground but if they are not (which is due to tight calf muscles), simply place a book or cushion for support. In time, the muscle will lengthen and your heels will touch the floor.

Once in the squatting position, the knees will be in the armpits and the head should be bent forward so you can see your feet. Your hands should not rest on the floor. You will feel a stretch in the spine. Do not force a stretch. This should be a comfortable position.

Relax in this position, breathing normally, for about two minutes. A gentle rocking back and forth can be beneficial. Then slowly raise yourself.

This exercise is designed to stretch and strengthen the leg muscles, increase energy flow, and promote mental calmness.

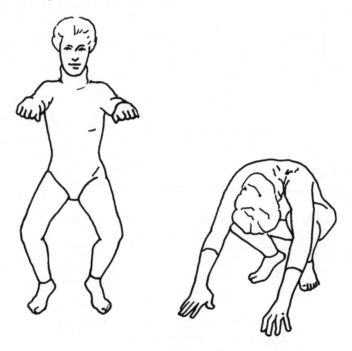

Spinal Rock

Sit on a well-padded, carpeted floor or an exercise mat. Place your hands on your thighs behind your knees and hold. Drop your chin to your chest. Slowly roll backward, pulling your knees toward you, with your spine curved forward. When you have finished rolling backward, push your feet forward to create momentum to rock forward. These movements should create a continuous, smooth, rocking motion of the body. Breathe normally and rock for about two minutes.

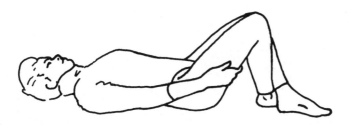

This is a stimulating exercise, increasing energy flow and mental clarity.

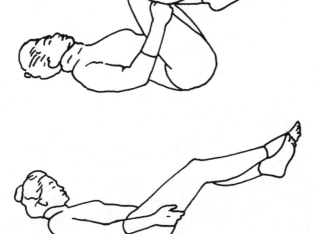

Natural Breathing

Lie on your back with your hands on your abdomen. Take a deep breath into the abdomen and feel the hands rise. Feel them lower as you exhale. The inhaling and exhaling should be slow and thorough, with a slight pause before the next inhale. Repeat 10 times.

This exercise has a calming and balancing effect on the mind and body.

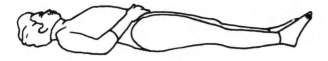

Fists in Calves

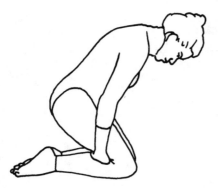

Kneel on a padded surface. Form fists and place them on your calves, behind your knees. Slowly lower the weight of your body as it pushes your fists into the calf muscle. Breathe slowly and focus on the calf area. For some people, this may produce some discomfort. If this is the case, use only as much weight as is comfortable and pause if necessary.

This exercise stimulates blood circulation.

Peaceful Sitting

Sit on a comfortable, padded floor. Place your feet flat in front of you and bring your heels as close as is comfortable to your buttocks. Your knees are up in front of you. Drop your chin to your chest as you relax your neck. Interlock your fingers across the back of your neck and allow your arms to hang. Relax and breathe slowly and naturally for as long as you like. You may choose to raise your head up, periodically, and outstretch your elbows with your hands still on your neck and be aware of your surroundings. Then, relax again with your head down.

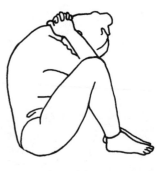

This is a very peaceful, relaxing exercise that is meant to be enjoyable and rejuvenating.

Recommended Reading

The Polarity Process: Energy as a Healing Art, Franklyn Sills (England: Element Books Limited, 1989).
Polarity Therapy: The Power That Heals, Alan Siegal, N.D. (San Leandro, California: Prism Press, 1987).

18

Reflexology

Reflexologists believe that the proper stimulation of reflex points can affect a particular organ, gland or area of the body to improve or alleviate many health problems. It also contributes to the health and harmony of the total person in a natural way.
—Hugh Burroughs & Mark Kastner,
Alternative Healing

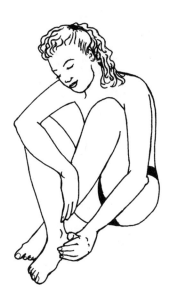

❧

For Health & Well-Being

Reflexology techniques use finger and hand pressure that is applied to specific areas (reflex points) on the feet and hands. These areas correspond to an organ, gland or area of the body. The pressure stimulates the reflex points and is believed to beneficially affect the corresponding body part. This encourages the body's natural ability to heal itself, bringing about better health and increased well-being. (The principles of reflexology are similar to those of acupressure.)

Reflexology was both named and perfected by Eunice Ingham in the 1930s. Ms. Ingham was a physiotherapist who used methods of "zone therapy" (certain areas of the body corresponding to other parts) popularized by Dr. William Fitzgerald for reducing pain. While working with zone therapy, she discovered methods that increased the therapeutic effects. She developed the Ingham Reflex Method of Compression Massage—later to be called Reflexology.

To explain Reflexology's effect on the body, Ms. Ingham said that it increases the circulation and raises the body vitality. As the vitality increases, nature has the strength to overcome and throw off the poisons in the system. Reflexology has been used successfully to enhance cardiovascular performance, boost the immune system, help shed extra pounds, increase energy, and relieve stress.

❧

For Skin Care

Reflexology can be used for skin care to increase the vitality of organs and glands that directly affect the condition of the skin. Specifically, these are the pituitary, the liver, the lungs, the adrenals, the kidneys, the intestinal tract, and the lymphatic system. Reflexology can improve dry, oily, or blemished skin and relieve stress that may be aggravating these conditions.

The technique: On each reflex point, press firmly and massage deeply with your thumb in a circular motion to the count of ten. Release the pressure slightly to the count of three and then repeat five times.

The Pituitary Gland

The pea-sized pituitary gland is located on the underside of the brain. It secretes hormones that are vital to life, monitors the activity of other hormone-producing glands, and balances the glandular functions in the body. Both hormones and glandular function have a significant impact on the skin, especially in the production of oil from the sebaceous glands.

The pituitary reflex point is located in the center of the pad on each big toe.

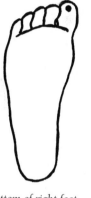

bottom of right foot   *bottom of left foot*

The Liver

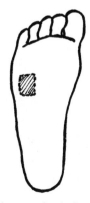

bottom of right foot

The liver is the largest internal organ, located on the right side, under the ribs. It is indispensable, performing more than 500 biochemical functions such as aiding digestion, filtering waste products, storing and releasing vitamins, and manufacturing vital compounds such as bile. Good liver function is especially important for skin that is blemished.

The liver reflex point is located on the right foot beneath the two last toes and about one-third of the way to the heel.

The Lungs

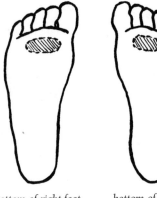

bottom of right foot   *bottom of left foot*

The right lung has three lobes and is slightly larger than the left lung, which has only two lobes. The lungs have no muscles of their own and are expanded and collapsed by the surrounding chest muscles. As we breathe, air enters the trachea, which divides into two bronchial tubes (one for each lung) and then into smaller branches. The lungs help to clean the air that we breathe as well as exchange carbon dioxide for oxygen. The oxygen is then circulated through the body by the bloodstream. Good lung function is especially important for the proper oxygenation of skin.

The reflex point for the lungs is located on both feet, on the ball of the foot, below the middle three toes.

The Adrenals

The adrenal glands are located on top of the kidneys and are about the size of a fingertip. They manufacture more than fifty different hormones or hormone-like chemicals that are crucial to body functions such as fat metabolism, water and mineral balance, and the reduction of inflammation. Adrenal glands are important for skin care to reduce the effects of stress and help control and calm blemishes.

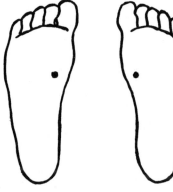

bottom of right foot   *bottom of left foot*

The reflex point for the adrenals is on both feet, is located at the base of the ball of the foot, in between the big toe and the next toe.

The Kidneys

The kidneys are bean-shaped organs about the size of a fist located behind the stomach at the level of the bottom edge of the back ribs. The kidneys clean and filter the blood and regulate mineral levels and water balance. This process produces urine—approximately two quarts every day. The condition of the kidneys is important for the skin to maintain optimum moisture balance and to clear blemishes.

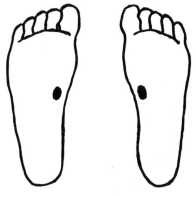

bottom of right foot   *bottom of left foot*

The reflex points of the kidneys are on both feet, located in the arch almost in the center but towards the inner edge.

The Intestines

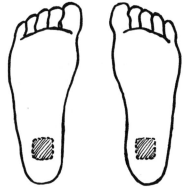

bottom of right foot   *bottom of left foot*

Part of the digestive system, the intestines are approximately twenty-six feet long, coiled in the abdomen. As food leaves the stomach, it enters the intestines, where it is processed into nutrients and water. Intestinal villi then absorb the nutrients and water to be used by the body. Good intestinal health is crucial for a clear and well-nourished complexion.

The intestinal reflex area is located on both feet, though the area is slightly different on each foot. It is centered on the foot, just above the heel and extends to the middle of the arch.

The Lymphatic System

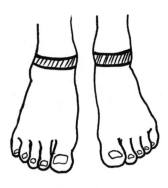

The lymphatic system is designed to clean, nourish, and protect the tissues and organs of the body and remove their waste products. The system includes the capillary network, the collecting vessels, and the lymph glands. Together, they distribute fluid and transport wastes. The lymph nodes are part of the body's defense system and produce antibodies to fight infection. The lymph system is very important for clearing blemishes.

The reflex areas for the lymphatic system are on the top side of both feet where the ankle joins the feet extending from the inner ankle bone to the outer.

NOTE: For corresponding reflex points on the hands, see page 93.

Recommended Reading

The Reflexology Workout, Stephanie Rick and Rita Aero (New York: Harmony Books, 1986).

Body Reflexology, Mildred Carter (New York: Parker Publishing Company, 1983).

19

Managing Stress

Stress is inherent in every healthy form of life; it is the
force exerted by any one thing against another. Stress is,
always has been, and always will be, a part of being alive.
—L. John Mason, Ph.D., Guide to Stress Reduction

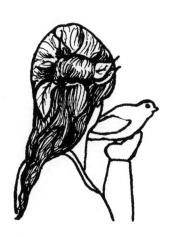

❧

For Health & Well-Being

S tress has become one of the major health concerns of our time. Stress can be mental, emotional, or physical and contributes to a variety of modern-day maladies. Stress from emotional causes is more likely to produce disease than stress from too much mental activity, or physical work. Heart disease, cancer, ulcers, high blood pressure, irritability, chronic fatigue, migraines, backaches, rashes, acne, and digestive disorders have all been linked to stress. What causes it? How does it affect us? The answers are subjective and personal—what causes stress for one person may not for another. Whatever the cause, when we are "stressed," we feel emotionally or physically threatened, and prolonged stress can make us ill. Learning and practicing stress reduction and management skills that induce a relaxation response may be one of the best ways to maintain good physical and mental health.

❧

For Skin Care

Stress can ruin our complexion. As described by Aveline Kushi, "Tension and anxiety cause the body to release androgens that activate oil-producing glands in the skin. The result is often an outbreak of acne, pimples or oily skin. Other hormones secreted in response to changes in moods and emotions influence such external features as the color, elasticity and tone of the skin, the circulation of blood to the capillaries below the skin and the formation of new skin and hair cells."[1]

Because of this relationship between stress and the complexion, it is important to learn stress management skills if you want your skin to look its best. Natural, alternative techniques offer a variety of ways to help us deal with the stress in our lives. Several methods are listed below and may remind you of—or introduce you to—available relief. If any interest you, it is recommended that you try one at a time so you will be aware of its effect in your life. Once you know how you react to a technique, it is possible to work in combination with others, as long as you introduce only one at a time.

Self-Help Techniques

Meditation

In relationship to stress (as opposed to a spiritual practice), meditation is a relaxation technique. It provides many benefits when practiced regularly. It can relax the body, rejuvenate the nervous system, clear and refine mental activity, and lower the blood pressure. Meditation is a technique of directed concentration that allows for deep mental and physical relaxation—even better than sleep. It awakens the intuition as well as positive, constructive tendencies, and most people experience a deep inner satisfaction. Meditation promotes a sense of well-being and an improved outlook on life and can lift minor depression. It increases energy because of the deep rest it allows and promotes mental peace with emotional calmness.

Technique #1

Find a quiet place. Sit upright in a comfortable position. Loosen any clothing that is tight or causing discomfort. Become aware of your natural pattern of breathing. Do not try to change it; simply observe it. Do this for twenty minutes. Do not overanalyze what you have just experienced. Do not judge it as a "good" or "bad" meditation.

Technique #2

Find a quiet place and sit upright in a comfortable position. Loosen any clothing that is too tight. Close your eyes. Think of a simple word that makes you feel good such as "om," "amen," or "peace." "Watch" your breathing and hear the word in your mind on the exhale of your breath. Do this for twenty minutes. Come out of your meditation slowly and gently, feeling revitalized.

Recommended Reading

How to Meditate, Laurence Le Shan (New York: Bantam Books, 1974).
How to Meditate, John Novak (Nevada City, CA: Crystal Clarity Publishers, 1989).
Sharing Silence, Gunilla Norris (New York: Bell Tower/ Crown Publishers, 1992).

Reflexology

Reflexology, as previously discussed in Chapter 18, can be used regularly for stress reduction or to provide some relief whenever you are feeling tense.

Reflexology on the Hands

Massage the base of the middle and ring fingers on the palm. This prompts the lungs to increase the blood's oxygen level, which will refresh and nurture the body. It helps to establish a regular, more relaxed breathing pattern.

Massaging the length of the front of the thumbs (the side where the nail is) encourages the spinal cord to soothe nerve responses.

Massaging the ball of the thumb stimulates the pituitary gland to cause a calming sensation.

Massaging the base of the thumb on the palm side encourages the thyroid and parathyroid glands to balance muscle tension, causing the body to relax.

Massaging the webbing between the thumb and forefinger helps to stimulate the kidneys, balancing fluid levels that affect blood pressure.

Reflexology on the Feet

Massaging the base of the four smaller toes on the top of the foot as well as on the sole of the foot prompts the lungs to increase the blood's oxygen level, which will refresh and nurture the body. It helps to establish a regular, more relaxed breathing pattern.

Massaging the outer edge of the foot along the big toe to the heel encourages the spinal cord to soothe nerve responses.

Massaging the arch of the foot (toward the side of the big toe) encourages the kidneys to balance fluid levels that affect blood pressure.

Massaging the ball of the big toe stimulates the pituitary gland to create a calming sensation.

(For more information and Recommended Reading, see Chapter 18, Reflexology.)

Bach Flower Remedies

Bach Flower Remedies are excellent for helping reduce the negative effects of too much stress in our lives. They can help to heal your mental attitude and allow you to get on with finding a solution to your problems because Dr. Bach felt that with hope, all things are possible. See Chapter 4, under "Alternatives Techniques for Blemished Skin," to learn more about Bach Flower Remedies. Refer also to the books suggested below.

Recommended Reading

The Bach Flower Remedies, Edward Bach, M.D. & F.J. Wheeler, M.D. (New Canaan, CT: Keats Publishing, 1979).

Bach Flower Therapy: Theory and Practice, Mechthild Scheffer (Rochester, VT Thorson Publishers Inc., 1987).

Flower Remedies Handbook, Donna Cunningham (New York: Sterling Publishing, 1992).

Nutrition and Supplements

Because nutrition plays such an important role in our physical and mental well-being, it also plays a role in managing stress. Your dietary habits can aggravate or relieve your stress levels. This includes *how* you eat, *when* you eat, *what* you eat, *where* you eat, and *why* you eat. Meals should be eaten slowly and chewed well.

You should not overeat because it overloads the digestion process. Do not eat during times of extreme emotional upset.

Foods should be varied, natural, and void of chemicals and additives. The body requires more high-quality, usable protein in times of stress. Foods to which you are allergic must be avoided, while eating healthy foods that you enjoy. You should have your meals in a pleasant environment, and lastly, you should only eat when you are hungry, not for an emotional need.

Some foods are known to raise anxiety and stress levels in sensitive individuals. Sugar and caffeine are the two major culprits. Sugar is so quickly absorbed into the bloodstream that the body thinks you are ready for "fight or flight." The heart beats faster, and the mind races in what is called the "sugar rush." Caffeine stimulates the nervous system, causing more rapid heartbeats and breathing. In addition, because caffeine is a diuretic, important water-soluble stress-preventing vitamins can be washed out of the body.

Certain vitamin and minerals are utilized by the body and depleted in times of stress, whether physical or emotional. Prolonged stress may warrant supplementation. The most important vitamins for protection against the harmful effects of stress are the B complex and vitamin C. The most important minerals are calcium, potassium, zinc, iron and magnesium.

For more information and Recommended Reading, review Chapter 16, "Nutrition."

Aromatherapy & Herbs

Used on a daily basis to encourage relaxation and peace of mind, aromatherapy is an effective and valuable practice that can alleviate stress. Essential oils especially good for this purpose are marjoram (in small amounts), chamomile (Roman), clary sage, bergamot, lavender, sandalwood, jasmine, and rose. When stress has caused lethargy, occasional use of stimulating essential oils such as rosemary or peppermint can be helpful. Essential oils can be used in warm baths, on a handkerchief that is sniffed frequently, or diluted in a base oil and massaged into the skin.

The herbal kingdom also provides us with valuable aids for stress management. Siberian ginseng is excellent for strengthening the body's resistance to the effects of stress. Relaxing herbs that calm the nervous system include valerian, hops, passion flower, skullcap, chamomile, and lavender. Herbs that can tone the nervous system are oats, St. Johnswort, and vervain. Herbs are easily used in hot or cold teas, and in foot baths or full baths.

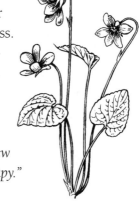

For more information and Recommended Reading, review Chapter 9, "Aromatherapy" and Chapter 13, "Herbal Therapy."

Breathing

As mentioned in Chapter 1, "A Checklist for Beautiful Skin: Breathe Well," breathing deeply and correctly can clear thinking, increase circulation, facilitate positive changes in moods and emotions, as well as tone the nervous system—enabling us to experience and enjoy life more fully. In fact, some stress reduction experts believe that deep breathing is the first step in learning to relax and unwind.

In breathing for relaxation, breathe in through the nose slowly and deeply—filling your lungs from the lowest part to the top. Hold the breath for a few seconds, then exhale through the mouth. By practicing deep breathing and controlling the breath, you can trigger a relaxation response in the body. When the breathing is slowed and deepened, the heart rate decreases and tension in the body can dissipate. Practice deep breathing on a daily basis, taking at least forty deep breaths a day.

Another method of breathing that can be used for relaxation and calming the nerves is called "color breathing," made popular by the late Linda Clark. In this method, simply sit in a quiet, meditative state (without disturbances) and breathe deeply, five or six times. Imagine that you are breathing in the color of sky blue, which is for relaxation and a sense of well-being. Then choose the color purple and breathe in—filling your whole body. Purple is for cleansing away physical and emotional disturbances.

Recommended Reading

Guide to Stress Reduction, L. John Mason, Ph.D. (Berkeley, CA: Celestial Arts, 1985).
Color Breathing, Linda Clark and Yvonne Martine (New York: Berkeley Publishing Corporation, 1976).

Visualization

Visualization is a technique that was made extremely popular by Shakti Gawain in her 1978 book, *Creative Visualization.* Visualization is used to change a mental or physical condition by creating a positive mental picture via the imagination. The body responds as if it were an actual experience, and profound changes can take place. Shakti states that creative visualization is the technique of using the imagination to create what you want in your life.

To use visualization as a anti-stress technique, sit down and take a few deep breaths. Imagine that you are calm, cool, and collected. This must be imagined in the here and now. (Not I will be. . .or I will learn to. . . .) Imagine all the wonderful things that happen when you are not stressed out. Imagine how your relationships with people are better. Imagine your work is pleasurable. Imagine how good you feel. See yourself as a relaxed person. The brain and body lodge these as actual experiences and they can bring about authentic change.

Recommended Reading

Creative Visualization, Shakti Gawain (Berkeley CA: Whatever Publishing, 1978).
Guide to Stress Reduction, L. John Mason, Ph.D. (Berkeley, CA: Celestial Arts, 1985).

A Collection of Stress-Releasing Ideas

1. Have a good cry. Tears can help relieve stress by ridding the body of potentially harmful chemicals produced in times of stress. Tears release ten-

sion and built-up anxiety and are the body's natural response to stress from many emotions such as fear, anger, love, joy, hurt feelings, or pain.

2. Learn to pray. Offering your troubles to a higher source can ease the strain.

3. Scream (but only where it won't scare someone). This is especially good to relieve pent-up anger. Good places to scream are in the shower, while you are driving (with the windows rolled up), or into your pillow.

4. Talk it out. Acknowledge your emotions, whether they be anger or fear or hate, and talk about what is troubling you so that the pressure does not build up.

5. Have some fun. Movies, books, visits to museums, crafts, or spectator sports can all take your mind off your stressful situation and provide relief.

6. Clear up clutter. Whether it is at home or at the job, clutter causes confusion, and confusion contributes to stress.

7. Take a walk, with no particular purpose or pace. Allow yourself to daydream.

8. Get a massage. It is well known that tension is stored in the body, especially in the muscles. A good massage can work some of those tensions away.

9. Laughter releases pent-up emotions and helps to get rid of painful feelings. During a good laugh, the body starts pumping adrenaline, the heart rate increases, the brain releases endorphins (natural pain killers), the lungs pump out carbon dioxide, the eyes cleanse themselves with tears, and the muscles relax and lose tension.

10. Next time you are frazzled, check your breathing. Chances are that it's shallow and rapid. Consciously take three slow, deep breaths and repeat every few minutes. This will immediately begin to discharge the stress.

11. A lot of tension builds up in the neck. Relax and stretch the neck muscles by dropping the head to the chest, looking one way and then the other. Massage the neck.

12. Shoulders are another place where tension is stored. Stretch and relax these muscles by shrugging your shoulders and then releasing. Massage.

13. Seclusion can be revitalizing. Set aside some time every day, even if it is just for a few minutes, to be totally alone in a peaceful environment.

14. Turn to your friends. An objective viewpoint may help to put things into perspective for you. Social support buffers stresses and can make them more tolerable.

15. Be present. Learn to appreciate the here and now and whatever you are currently doing. Try to stop worrying about the past and future.

16. Use empty times. While you are waiting or standing in line, practice relaxing and breathing deeply—from head to toe.

17. Exercise is a natural stress reducer. It is hard to be uptight or tense when you are physically tired.

18. Practice giving and receiving a hug every day. It's good for you.

19. Music was an integral part of ancient Egyptian medicine, and the Greeks also believed that music restored health to both body and soul. It is believed that certain types of music (generally soft and soothing tones) cause the body to release endorphins, bringing about pain relief and relaxation. Listening to your favorite music can be uplifting and stress-reducing.

20. Time management is essential. Schedule your day with breaks and free time, in addition to your regular responsibilities.

21. Reward yourself. If you have handled a stressful situation well or gotten through one unscathed, take yourself out to dinner or buy something new.

22. Count your blessings. If you stop and think about it, there are probably many things going right in your life.

23. Keep a dream diary. You do not have to be able to formally interpret your dreams, but it can be valuable to remember them and the feelings they catalyzed. Keep a pad and pencil by the bed. When you wake, write

down any part or all of a dream that you had during the night. Dreams can bring your attention to feelings you may not be consciously aware of and can reduce their stress.

24. Don't take on too much. There is a limit to everyone's capacity. Trying to do too much is very stressful. Learn to say "no" when appropriate and better schedule your time.

25. Persistent mental and physical symptoms of stress should be checked out with your doctor. There may be a medical problem.

26. Get enough sleep. Your night's sleep is the time to recover from the day's activities. If you awake refreshed and ready to go, you are getting the amount and quality you need. If not, you may need to change your sleep habits to ensure that you get the amount you need.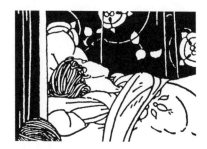

27. Learn to accept what you cannot change.

28. Do something good for others. It gets your mind off yourself and is one way to achieve social connectedness that can counteract the stress of feeling lonely or isolated.

29. When you are stressed out, get a piece of paper and write down, in great detail, the scope of the problem and how you would like it solved. Once everything that you have on your mind is on the paper you can throw it away because you have gotten it out of your system.

30. Schedule a time every day that is your "personal time" and do something that relaxes you or that you really enjoy.

31. If being fatigued is causing stress and making you short-tempered, try a cat-nap during the day—ten or fifteen minutes is enough to provide relief without upsetting the nighttime sleep cycle.

32. Eliminate caffeinated drinks from your diet. They can increase muscle tension and make you feel nervous and stressed out.

33. Keep life's events in perspective. There is a wonderful expression from Robert Eliot's book, *Is it Worth Dying For?* He says that there are basically two rules to stress management. 1) Don't sweat the small stuff and 2) It's all small stuff.

34. If you are feeling tense at the end of the day, take a nice, warm, relaxing bath or shower.

35. Consider changing the situations in your life that are causing you stress.

36. Spend some time connecting with nature. Take a walk in a park. Visit a flower nursery or a beautiful garden.

37. Spend some time with a pet, especially if it is your own. Slow-paced animals have a way of relaxing us and they also relieve feelings of isolation.

38. Develop your spirituality. People who believe in a higher power can keep life's difficulties in perspective.

Glossary of Terms

Allergens are substances that cause an exaggerated or pathological reaction when they come in contact with body tissue by skin absorption, ingestion or inhalation.

Antiseptics inhibit the growth of germs and microorganisms such as bacteria, yeast, and mold.

Astringents have a tightening, constricting action on the skin.

Anti-Oxidants are substances that inhibit oxidation. The term anti-oxidant is frequently linked with the term "free radicals" because anti-oxidants protect living cells from free radical damage. Anti-oxidants such as vitamin A (including beta carotene), vitamin C, vitamin E, bioflavonoids, selenium, zinc, ginkgo biloba, ginseng, pycnogenol, and aloe vera can help prevent free radical damage and premature aging of the skin. It is thought that these substances may be more effective for the skin when applied externally than if used internally, because a direct application will not be used elsewhere in the body.

Biodegradable means that a substance can be broken down by microorganisms to its organic components.

Creams are a cosmetic formulation that is the result of an emulsion (see) of water and oil. The water softens and moisturizes the skin while the oil protects it from the environment and moisture loss. Creams are thicker in consistency than lotions.

Emollients are conditioners that soothe, soften, and protect the skin.

Emulsions are the suspension of either water-in-oil or oil-in-water. This suspension prevents the water and oil from separating.

Emulsifiers enable an oil to be dispersed in water or water to be dispersed in oil. (Normally, water and oil do not mix.)

Enzymes are complex proteins that act as catalysts for biochemical reactions in the body.

Essential Oils are volatile oils obtained from a variety of plant parts (leaf, flower, bark, root, stem, or seed), usually by distillation.

Exfoliants are used to encourage the sloughing off of old, dead skin cells from the surface of the skin.

Extracts result from combining a soluble substance with a solvent such as an herb in alcohol.

Free Radicals are molecular particles—unstable atoms that have an unpaired electron. When trying to stabilize, they steal another atom's electron. As the first becomes stabilized, the other then has an unpaired electron, becoming a free radical. . .and it continues as a chain reaction. Although the body is capable of handling some free radicals, the amount created in the body by today's environment may be overwhelming. Over-exposure to the ultraviolet rays of the sun, infections or disease, physical or mental exhaustion, hormonal imbalance, pollution, alcohol, fatty foods, and cigarette smoke all contribute to the formation of free radicals. Free radicals increase oxidation, damage cells, and promote degenerative changes associated with disease and aging. The skin reflects this onslaught of free radical damage in the form of dryness, wrinkling, loss of elasticity, and "age spots."

Humectants are ingredients that attract and hold moisture to the skin. Because moisture plays such an important role in the condition of the skin—keeping it moist and supple, preventing wrinkles, and promoting softness and smoothness—humectants are important ingredients, especially in moisturizers.

Hypoallergenic means that a product or an ingredient is *less* likely to cause an allergic reaction than similar products or ingredients. An allergic reaction is still possible.

Irritants are substances that cause an adverse reaction to the skin such as itching, blisters, redness, or swelling.

Lotions are a cosmetic formulation that is the result of an emulsion. The water softens and moisturizes the skin while the oil provides a film on the surface skin to protect it from the environment and moisture loss. Lotions are more fluid than a cream.

Ph is an abbreviation for potential hydrogen. It represents a scale from 0 to 14, and is used to measure the alkalinity or acidity of a solution. 7.0 is considered neutral. Below 7.0 is acidic and above 7.0 is alkaline.

Preservatives are used in cosmetics to prevent rancidity and the contamination of molds, fungi, viruses, and bacteria.

Sensitizers are substances that cause the development of skin irritations. A sensitizer may cause a reaction anywhere on the body—not only where it was applied.

Bibliography

Acupressure's Potent Points, Michael Reed Gach (New York: Bantam Books, 1990).

Advanced Professional Skin Care, Peter T. Pugliese, M. D. (Bernville, PA: APSC Publishing, 1991).

The Aida Grey Beauty Book, Aida Grey (New York: J. B. Lippingcott Company, 1979).

Alternative Healing, Hugh Burrows and Mark Kastner, Dipl.Ac. (La Mesa, CA: Halcyon Publishing, 1993).

Aromatherapy: An A to Z, Patricia Davis (England: C. W. Daniel Company Limited, 1988).

Aromatherapy: Answers to the Most Commonly Asked Questions, Michael Scholes (Los Angeles: Aromatherapy Seminars, 1993).

The Aromatherapy Book, Jeanne Rose (Berkeley, CA: North Atlantic Books, 1992).

Aromatherapy For Common Ailments, Shirley Price (New York: Simon and Schuster, 1991).

Aromatherapy: The Complete Guide to Plant and Flower Essences for Health and Beauty, Daniele Ryman (New York: Bantam Books, 1991).

Aromatherapy For Women, Maggie Tisserand (New York: Thorsons Publishers, 1985).

Aromatherapy: To Heal and Tend the Body, Robert Tisserand (Santa Fe, NM: Lotus Press, 1988).

Aromatherapy Workbook, Marcel Lavabre (Rochester, VT: Healing Arts Press, 1990).

The Art of Aromatherapy, Robert Tisserand (New York: Inner Traditions International Limited, 1977).

The Art of Breathing, Nancy Zi (New York: Bantam Books, 1986).

Ayurveda: The Science of Self-Healing, Dr. Vasant Lad (Santa Fe, NM: Lotus Press, 1984).

The Bach Flower Remedies, Edward Bach, M. D. and F. J. Wheeler (New Canaan, CT: Keats Publishing, Inc., 1979).

Bach Flower Therapy: Theory and Practice, Mechthild Scheffer (Rochester, VT: Thorsons Publishers, 1987).

The Bath Book, Gregory and Beverly Frazier (San Francisco: Troubador Press, 1973).

Body Reflexology, Mildred Carter (New York: Parker Publishing Company, 1983).

Breathing: The ABCs, Carola H. Speads (San Francisco: Harper Colophon Books, 1978).

Color Your Life, Howard and Dorothy Sun (New York: Ballantine Books, 1992).

The Compass in Your Nose & Other Astonishing Facts About Humans, Marc McCutcheon (Los Angeles, Jeremy P. Tarcher, Inc., 1989).

Complete Aromatherapy Handbook, Susanne Fischer-Rizze (New York: Sterling Publishing Company, 1990).

The Complete Book of Essential Oils and Aromatherapy, Valerie Ann Worwood (San Rafael, CA: New World Library, 1991).

The Complete Book of Water Therapy, Dian Dincin Buchman (New York: E. P. Dutton, 1979).

The Complete Herbal Guide to Natural Health & Beauty, Dian Dincin Buchman (New York: Doubleday & Company, 1973).

A Consumer's Dictionary of Cosmetic Ingredients, Ruth Winter (New York: Crown Publishers, Inc., 1989).

Color Breathing, Linda Clark & Yvonne Martin (New York: Berkeley Publishing Corporation, 1976).

Creative Visualization, Shakti Gawain (Berkeley, CA: Whatever Publishing, 1978).

Culpeper's Color Herbal, edited by David Potterton (New York: Sterling Publishing Company, Inc.,1983).

Diet for Natural Beauty, Aveline Kushi (New York, Japan Publications, Inc., 1991).

The Doctors' Vitamin and Mineral Encyclopedia, Sheldon Saul Hendler, M.D., Ph.D.(New York: Simon and Schuster, 1990).

Dr. Braly's Optimum Health Program, James Braly, M. D. (New York: Times Books, 1985).

Enchanting Scents, Monika Junemann (Wilmot, WI: Lotus Light Shangra-la, 1988).

The Encyclopaedia of Essential Oils, Julia Lawless (Rockport, MA: Element Books, 1992).

Everybody's Guide to Homeopathic Medicines, Stephen Cummings & Dana Ullman (Los Angeles: Jeremy P. Tarcher, Inc., 1984).

Flower Essences and Vibrational Healing, Gurudas (San Rafael: Cassandra Press, 1989).

Flower Remedies Handbook, Donna Cunningham (New York: Sterling Publishing Co., 1992).

Food and Healing, Annemarie Colbin (New York: Balantine Books, 1986).

The Grosset Encyclopedia of Natural Medicine, Robert Thomson (New York: Grosset & Dunlap, 1980).

Guide to Stress Reduction, L. John Mason, Ph. D. (Berkeley, CA: Celestial Arts, 1985).

Hands, Linda Rose (Woodstock, NY: The Overlook Press, 1985).

The Healing Clay, Michel Abehsera (New York: Swan House Publishing, 1977).

The Healing Herbs of Edward Bach, Julian and Martine Barnard (Great Britain: Ashgrove Press, 1988).

The Healing Foods, Patricia Hausmann & Judith Benn Hurley (Emmaus, PA: Rodale Press, 1989).

The Healing Power of Color, Betty Wood (Rochester, VT: Destiny Books, 1992).

Healing with Whole Foods, Paul Pitchford (Berkeley, CA: North Atlantic Books, 1993).

Health, Youth, and Beauty Through Color Breathing, Linda Clark & Yvonee Martine (New York: Berkeley Publishing Corporation, 1976).

Healthy Healing, Linda G. Rector-Page, N. D., Ph. D. (Healthy Healing Publications, 1992).

The Herb Book, John Lust (New York: Bantam Books, 1974).

The Herbal Handbook, David Hoffman (Rochester, VT: Healing Arts Press, 1987).

Herbal Medicine, Dian Dincin Buchman (New York: David McKay Company, 1979).

Holistic Aromatherapy, Ann Berwick (St. Paul, MN: Llewellyn Publication, 1994).

How to Meditate, John Novak (Nevada City, CA: Crystal Clarity Publishers, 1989).

Jeanne Rose's Kitchen Cosmetics, Jeanne Rose (San Francisco: Panjandrum/Aris Books, 1978).

Lilias, Yoga & Your Life, Lilias Folan (New York: MacMillan Publishing, 1981).

Liz Earle's Natural Beauty, Liz Earle (London: Vermilion, 1993).

Magical Aromatherapy, Scott Cunningham (St. Paul, MN: Llewellyn Publications, 1989).

Massage: The Oriental Method, Katsusuke Serizawa, M. D. (Tokyo: Japan Publications, 1972).

Modern Esthetics, Henry J. Gambino (New York: Milady Publishing Company, 1992).

Modern Magic of Natural Healing with Water Therapy, J. V. Cerney (New York: Parker Publishing Company, Inc., 1975).

Natural Health, Natural Medicine, Andrew Weil, M. D. (Boston: Houghton Mifflin Co., 1990).

New Beauty: Acupressure Face Lift, Lindsay Wagner & Robert Klein (Englewood Cliffs, NJ: Prentice Hall, 1987).

Nontoxic, Natural, & Earthwise, Debra Lynn Dadd (Los Angeles, Jeremy P. Tarcher, 1990).

The Pendulum Kit, Sig Lonegran (New York: Simon and Schuster, 1990).

The Polarity Process: Energy as a Healing Art, Franklyn Sills (Great Britain: Element Books, 1989).

Polarity Therapy: The Power that Heals, Alan Siegel, N. D. (San Leandro, CA: Prism Press, 1987).

Positive Living and Health, editors of *Prevention* magazine and the Center for Positive Living (Emmaus, PA: Rodale Press, 1990).

Practical Aromatherapy, Shirley Price (London: Thorsons Publishers Limited, 1983).

The Practice of Aromatherapy, Jean Valnet, M. D. (Rochester, VT: Healing Arts Press, 1980).

Prescription for Nutritional Healing, James F. Balch, M.D. & Phyllis A. Balch, C.N.C. (New York: Avery Publishing Group, 1990).

The Reflexology and Color Therapy Workbook, Pauline Wills (Great Britain: Element Books, 1992).

The Reflexology Workout, Stephanie Rick & Rita Aero (New York: Harmony Books, 1986).

Sharing Silence, Gunilla Norris (New York: Bell Tower/Crown Publishers, 1992).

Shirley Price's Aromatherapy Workbook, Shirley Price (San Francisco: Thorsons, 1993).

Skin Care and Cosmetic Ingredients Dictionary, Natalia Michalun (New York: Milady Publishing Company, 1994).

The Smoker's Book of Health, Tom Ferguson (New York: Putnam and Sons, 1987).

Standard Textbook of Cosmetology, edited by Israel Rubinstein (New York: Milady Publishing, 1981).

Stretching, Bob Anderson (Bolinas, CA: Shelter Publications, 1980).

Subtle Aromatherapy, Patricia Davis (England: C. W. Daniel Company Limited, 1991).

Take Care of Yourself: The Healthtrac Guide to Medical Care, James F. Fries, M. D. & Donald M. Vickery, M. D. (Menlo Park, CA: Addison-Wesley Publishing Co., 1993).

The 12-Minute Total Body Workout, Joyce L. Vedral (New York: Warner Books, 1989).

Vital Oils, Liz Earle (London: Vermilion, 1992).

The Way of Herbs, Michael Tierra, C. A., N. D. (New York: Washington Square Press, 1983).

Webster's Ninth New Collegiate Dictionary (Springfield, MA: Merriam-Webster Inc., 1986).

The Yoga of Herbs: An Ayurvedic Guide to Herbal Medicine, Dr. David Frawley and Dr. Vasant Lad (Santa Fe, NM: Lotus Press, 1986).

Your Body and How it Works, J. D. Ratcliff (Readers Digest Press, 1975).

Notes

Chapter 1: The Checklist for Beautiful Skin

1. J.D. Ratcliff, *Your Body and How it Works* (Readers Digest Press, 1976), 57.
2. Peter T. Pugliese, M. D., *Advanced Professional Skin Care* (Bernville, PA: APSC Publishing, 1991), 59.
3. J. D. Ratcliff, *Your Body and How it Works* (Readers Digest Press and Delacorte Press, 1976), 55.
4. Henry J. Gambino, *Modern Esthetics* (Albany, NY: Milady Publishing Company, 1992), 99.
5. Peter T. Pugliese, M.D., "Physiology of the Skin: Sun's Effect on the Skin," *Skin, Inc.* June 1989): 42, 90.
6. Lynn Gagnon, "Save Lives: Teach Sun Protection from Birth," *Dermascope* (March/April 1991): 56.
7. Bruce I. White, M.D., FA. C. S., "Cigarette Smoking Causes Aging of the Skin," *Dermascope* (September/October 1989): 14.
8. Bruce I. White, M.D., FA. C. S., "Cigarette Smoking Causes Aging of the Skin," *Dermascope* (September/October 1989): 14.
9. Betty Franklin, "Catching Up," *Let's Live* (January 1988): 80.
10. Cathy Sears, "Updates," American Health (June 1990): 30.
11. Dr. Arnold Pike, D. C., "Is Your Life Going Up in Smoke?," *Let's Live* (October 1991): 26.

12. Usha Lee McFarling, "Are you Sleep Deprived?," *Natural Health* (January/February 1994): 64.

Chapter 2: What is Your True Skin Type?

1. "Accutane Warning Reemphasized," *FDA Consumer* (June 1984): 3.

Chapter 4: Skin Care Programs

1. Lee Ockey, "Sensitive Skin & Cosmetics," *Dermascope* (July/August 1991): 88.
2. Jane Bell, personal communication, 1995.

Chapter 5: Skin Care for the Body

1. Suzanne Chazin, "Splendor in the Bath," American Health (October 1990): 58.

Chapter 6: Natural Ingredients for Skin Care

1. Sheldon Saul Hendler, M. D., Ph. D., *The Doctors' Vitamin and Mineral Encyclopedia* (New York: Simon and Shuster, 1990), 37.

Chapter 10: Ayurveda

1. Hugh Burrows & Mark Kastner, *Alternative Healing* (La Mesa, CA: Halcyon Publishing, 1993), 28.
2. Janaki, personal communication, May 1995. I am indebted for her valuable information about Ayurvedic aesthetics.

Chapter 11: Color Therapy

1. Hugh Burrows & Mark Kastner, *Alternative Healing* (La Mesa, CA: Halcyon Publishing, 1993), 62.
2. Hugh Burrows & Mark Kastner, *Alternative Healing* (La Mesa, CA: Halcyon Publishing, 1993), 63.

3. Ruth Strock, director of The Color Research Institute, San Francisco, personal communication, 1989.
4. Hugh Burrows & Mark Kastner, *Alternative Healing* (La Mesa, CA: Halcyon Publishing, 1993), 63.
5. Ruth Strock, director of The Color Research Institute, San Francisco, personal communication, 1989.

Chapter 13: Herbal Therapy

1. Hugh Burrows & Mark Kastner, *Alternative Healing* (La Mesa, CA: Halcyon Publishing, 1993), 107.

Chapter 14: Hydrotherapy

1. Dian Dincin Buchman, *The Complete Book of Water Therapy* (New York: E. P. Dutton, 1979), 3.

Chapter 15: Massage

1. Hugh Burrows & Mark Kastner, *Alternative Healing* (La Mesa, CA: Halcyon Publishing, 1993), 156.

Chapter 16: Nutrition

1. James Braly, M. D., *Dr. Braly's Optimum Health Program* (New York: Times Books, 1985), 25.

Chapter 19: Managing Stress

1. Aveline Kushi, *Diet for Natural Beauty* (New York: Japan Publications. Inc., 1991), 105.

Index